CANNABIS GROWING

A COMPLETE AND SIMPLE GUIDE ON GROWING MEDICAL MARIJUANA AT HOME

BY

Doreen Weed

The trademarks used are without any consent, and the publication of the trademark is without permission or backing by the trademark owner. All trademarks and brands inside this book are for clarifying purposes only and are the owned by the owners themselves, not affiliated with this document.

As we addressed in this book, new practical seeds (ready to be planted and to produce another plant) will develop in the colas of the female plants in the two to about four months after they have been pollinated by a close male plant. The pistils on the seedpods may change hues before the cases burst and the new seeds will be dissipated to the topsoil beneath. However, this isn't the best way to get tightly to pot seeds so as to proceed with the strain.

You can abstain from growing new unidentified male seeds and proceed with the cannabis life cycle of your best plants through a procedure known as *sensimilla cloning*. You can become new, hereditarily indistinguishable variants of your preferred strains a seemingly endless amount of time after year, by cutting a part of at least four creeps from your best plant and planting it in establishing arrangement.

Summarizing The Lifecycle Of The Cannabis Plant

Splash your pot seeds in water or in a paper towel to grow the taproot that will secure into your topsoil and develop into seedlings. Continue checking the plant's hubs during the vegetative stage to guarantee that you don't have any undesirable male plants among your crop.

On the off chance that you do discover male plants, make certain to isolate them from the female plants. The cannabis plant will keep on vegetating until it starts to get less light from characteristic or fake sources. This will trigger its flowering stage.

Focus on the shades of the slight hairs or guns and on the shade of the leaders of the trichomes in order to decide the correct minute to trim and gather your plant. Hang the wet weed buds up in a cool, dull, dry space with low moistness for around seven days.

Before you can make the most of your wonderful new buds, you will have to fix them in glass artisan containers for one to three weeks, guaranteeing to open them once every day.

In case you are keen on growing a future arrangement of buds, you can proceed with the marijuana development cycle by enabling a male plant to fertilize a female one into developing seeds, with which you can explore different avenues regarding, or you can cut a branch from your preferred plant and spot it in attaching answer for clone it, season after season.

That is Biology. Shouldn't something be said about Technology?

In this book, we have concentrated on the science of the developing pant of marijuana, from seed to gather. In any case, there is progressively engaged with delivering your own cannabis crop rather than simply realizing how to distinguish the different phases of plant development.

An effective develop additionally requires a touch of innovation, regardless of whether you are becoming your weed outside. To get within scoop on that side of the challenge, look at *How To Grow Weed: The Organic Way*. At that point you can begin to develop it!

TABLE OF CONTENTS

The craft of cannabis development is advancing quickly, especially thanks to the developing acknowledgment of weed. But also thanks to the *open doors* of a directed market to a blasting industry. As increasingly potential purchasers, specialists, business visionaries and trailblazers direct their concentration toward cannabis, new and creative techniques to improve development are being found. Here at Grown Rogue, we are persistently searching for approaches to limit our characteristic asset use and exercise our ecological impression. For the reasons of this presentation, we will feature the three most well known develop strategies:

The Three Main Growing Environments for Cannabis

- **OUTDOOR**

Outdoor cannabis development depends on the accessible daylight during the evolving seasons, during which the plant is presented to the full range of light accessible in nature for that season. Outdoor cultivators experience a more extended development cycle and ordinarily just gather once per year.

Developing cannabis outdoors opens a crop to the components, offering regular light and fundamentally diminishing expenses, for cultivators. With no fake lights or fans required, power may just be required for water system.

While presentation to a common habitat is useful for plants, introduction to cruel ecological conditions may display deterrents to an outdoor crop. Downpour, bugs, intrusive plants (thorn, for example), creatures, and extraordinary weather conditions are for the most part potential crop executioners. Outdoor development additionally restricts cultivators' authority over natural hybrid from the close fields. To put it plainly, your kindred rancher's pesticides could wind up being your pesticides on the off chance that they are not expertly applied.

Outdoor cannabis cultivation while Indoor commonly directions the more significant expense in a dispensary. Most cannabis specialists will reveal you that a plant developed under the sun and presented to the full range of light, profiting by the environment, is the manner in which nature planned. Okay rather eat a strawberry picked from my natural nursery, or one become under a warmth light in a sterile domain? Using the sun, soil, and downpour to develop likewise implies that beginning an outdoor nursery is essentially more affordable than an evenhanded indoor activity.

Developing outdoors is not without its troubles. On the off chance that you profit by the amicableness gives, you likewise need to take the terrible. Wild creatures, storms, early ice, or a bunch of bugs that can influence a develop activity are constantly a potential risk. The way that outdoor develop activities just have one yield a year, implies any of those outside components can destroy everything for a nursery. At Grown Rogue, we do all that we can to relieve those dangers in our outdoor nurseries to furnish Oregon with top-rack, natural cannabis.

- **GREENHOUSE**

Developing cannabis in a greenhouse offers the free daylight of an outdoor develop, yet with far more prominent natural control. Greenhouses enable producers to control characteristic light with a power outage conceal or comparative rooftop covering framework. Greenhouses likewise offer the choice to add electrical lighting to enhance daylight on overcast days and an additional layer of security from creatures, vermin, and extraordinary natural changes.

One of the drawbacks to greenhouse development is the forthright cost required to have such a structure. Greenhouses extend from brief structures made of plastic and PVC pipe to perpetual structures that enable cultivators to control each natural angle and use propelled development strategies, including light hardship.

A risk in greenhouse developing is that nuisances can spread inside the encased condition at a quicker rate. Security against ecological hybrid is additionally constrained relying upon the kind of greenhouse structure.

Greenhouses offer the capacity to control light introduction, utilize supplemental lighting, if *Mother Nature* is not giving enough, and keep the atmosphere stable like indoor activities. Since the requirement for fake lighting is decreased, greenhouse tasks are commonly less expensive than developing indoors. However, as indoor tasks, greenhouses help to moderate introduction to the components making yields more reliable than outdoor activities.

- **INDOOR**

Indoor developing is normally performed in a distribution center setting, which requires counterfeit lighting and the utilization of cooling and dehumidification frameworks. The goal of an indoor develop is to emulate the outdoor components, encouraging plant development while keeping up full power over each natural parameter. The significant drawback of indoor developing is the high forthright and repeating costs that accompany the facilitiy, hardware, water, power, and different utilities.

Indoor cannabis cultivation chances are, on the off chance that you stroll into any dispensary, the normal cost per gram of indoor cannabis will be somewhere in the range of 15% – half higher than its outdoor partner. Indoor developed bloom will, in general, look all the more tastefully unblemished, have higher THC levels, and phenomenal fragrance and flavor profiles. By removing the bloom from the components and into a controlled situation, cultivators *kill* mileage on buds until they are being dealt with and relieved while, at the same time, they give the strain the definite atmosphere conditions it requires for most extreme yield. When a strain's subtleties are made sense of, the measure of cycles an indoor cultivator can create in a schedule year dwarves the one reap outdoor yields.

Atmosphere control frameworks can cost a fortune making indoor activities hard for most to begin at a scale. With outdoor, there is not a need to control temperature, lighting, CO_2 creation, or dampness. While new lighting is being grown consistently and the range indoor lights can cover is improving, there is no arrangement that matches the one of a kind range of light the sun gives.

Despite you are developing indoors it does not mean your plants aren not in danger for similar nuisances. While counteractive action in a directed situation is hypothetically simpler, when nuisances do show up, indoor activities do not have the assistance from nature they would have in outdoor activity; wasps, ants, and ladybugs all assistance to moderate parasite pervasions. It is imperative to recall that indoor, with its numerous cycles and controlled condition, guarantees we can give quality cannabis all throughout the entire year.

THINGS NEEDED FOR INDOOR

An indoor arrangement basically implies reproducing outdoor conditions in a controlled situation, one where a quality light is your closest companion and most significant part.

The main thing is on the off chance that you have a terrible light, it's simply not going to turn out incredible. High-wattage lights can be really modest on sites like Amazon . Great quality *high power release* or HID light that is vitality in order to develop the plant. For the flowering stage, a red-orange light is required, so a high weight sodium light, another sort of HID light, is convenient. Other lighting choices incorporate glaring lights (despite they are less effective) and LED lights, which can be exorbitant. A little tent (one that is two-by-four, three-by-three, or four-by-four feet) is likewise key to both keeping up the correct conditions and shielding the pot scent from barging in into the remainder of your home. Putting your arrangement in a spot with simple access to natural air that is likewise cool and dry. A fan is important for airflow. A carbon channel likewise helps expel that outstanding smell from getting away from the tent.

Contingent upon the amount you're willing to rampage spend, an invert assimilation framework can give you filtered water for your plants, despite the fact that spring water likewise works in case you are another specialist hoping to spare some money.

Basic supplement programs — versus a multi-bottle supplement framework — can likewise accommodate a decent develop for fledglings. Producers can go whichever way on engineered or natural supplements in any case if the develop is indoors or outside.

For a further developed arrangement, a dehumidifier and a forced air system can be helpful, but it is depending on the situation. By and large, a straightforward indoor apparatus could interfere with you two or three hundred dollars, the specialists state.

MARIJUANA'S HISTORY: HOW ONE PLANT SPREAD THROUGH THE WORLD

From the destinations where ancient trackers and gatherers lived, to antiquated China and Viking ships, cannabis has been utilized over the world for a very long time, and another report displays the medication's beautiful history.

In the report, writer Barney Warf depicts how cannabis utilize started a great many years back in Asia, and has since discovered its approach to numerous sides of the World, in the long run spreading to South and North America.

"Generally, it was broadly utilized for medication and profound purposes" said Warf, a teacher of topography at the University of Kansas, in Lawrence. For instance, the Vikings and medieval Germans utilized cannabis for diminishing agony during labor and for toothaches, he said.

"The possibility this is an underhanded medication is an ongoing development and the way that it is unlawful is a recorded peculiarity" said Warf. Marijuana has been legitimate in numerous locales of the world for the greater part of its history.

Nowadays it appears Wall Street has high trusts in the blooming cannabis industry, with marijuana stocks quickly picking up footing. Tilray (TLRY - Get Report) , the principal marijuana IPO in the United States, has been having a prime in the market, with one of the most amazing sessions recently that saw the stock shoot up over 90% before shutting lower. Furthermore, with an expected valuation of around 24 billion dollars, cannabis is never again a joke on The Street.

As different organizations like Coca-Cola deal with getting a bit of the pot pie, it appears the influx of endorsement for cannabis-based organizations and IPOs won't be halted.

History of Marijuana

The marijuana plant has its beginnings as a therapeutic plant a great many years back (numerous reports are followed back to Chinese Emperor Shen Nung in 2727 B.C.), and it was generally utilized by 500 B.C. in Asia. The plant, called *cannabis sativa*, supposedly experienced across the board use in an assortment of societies, including Indians, Muslims, Persians and the ancient Greeks and Romans.

Early employments of marijuana were to a great extent therapeutic, and it was utilized to treat things like aggravation, intestinal sickness, gout, discouragement, queasiness, as a soporific and even to stifle sexual wants. In any case, there is proof that a few societies utilized the psychoactive part of marijuana (THC) for customs or strict functions.

Marijuana was likely brought to North America by the Spanish in the late 1500s, and early settlements in the United States additionally developed marijuana and utilized hemp for an assortment of uses, for instance, utilizing the strands of the hemp plant to make paper, rope and different items.

Timetable of Marijuana

While marijuana has been being used both recreationally and restoratively for a large number of years, ongoing hundreds of years have seen a turbulent turn in the plant's lawfulness and history. From its disallowance in the mid 1930s to its moderate sanctioning over certain countries in the United States, cannabis has stayed a hotly debated issue of discussion. Yet its future currently appears to be encouraging as a developing business sector.

Marijuana in the United States

In the United States, early homesteaders developed hemp (a cannabis plant) frequently for use in materials or even things like making rope. By the 1600s, ranchers in states like Virginia, Massachusetts and Connecticut were developing the plant. It has even been proposed that Thomas Jefferson and George Washington developed hemp on their plantations.

Racial Undertones

During the 19th century *cannabis* was only used to allude to the plant. Nonetheless, when against Mexican feeling in the United States started to ascend in the mid 20th century, the term was changed to *marijuana* to cause to notice the medication's utilization by Mexicans (and along these lines endeavor to convey a negative implication).

Some basic speculations about the racial hints of the shame against cannabis flow around the administration partner marijuana use with perilous, desperate inclinations expedited by *locoweed* - Mexican cannabis. This disgrace, joined with the rising racial strains against ethnic minorities, added to expanding government guideline of the medication.

Truth be told, in an article entitled *More Reefer Madness*, The Atlantic clarified the probable racial starting points of the denial of marijuana.

"The political change in Mexico that finished in the Revolution of 1910 prompted an influx of Mexican migration to states all through the American Southwest. The biases and fears that welcomed these laborer outsiders additionally reached out to their conventional methods for inebriation: smoking marijuana. Cops in Texas asserted that marijuana induced rough violations, excited a desire for blood and gave its clients superhuman quality. Rumors spread that Mexicans were dispersing this executioner weed to clueless American schoolchildren. Mariners and West Indian settlers carried the act of smoking marijuana to port urban communities along the Gulf of Mexico. In New Orleans, paper articles connected the medication with African-Americans, jazz performers, whores, and black market whites. The Marijuana Menace, as portrayed by hostile to sedate campaigners, was embodied by second rate races and social freaks" revealed The Atlantic revealed a 1997 issue.

Moreover, the notorious statement by Harry Anslinger, one of the pioneers of the restriction, peruses that *"There are 100,000 absolute marijuana smokers in the U.S. Their Satanic music, jazz and swing is a result of using marijuana. This marijuana makes white ladies look for sexual relations with Negroes, performers and any others."*

While the racial language may have since to a great extent dispersed, The Guardian announced for the current year that in 2016, six hundred thousands cannabis-related captures occurred, with the vast dominant part influencing minorities. What is more, after the 2016 presidential political race, Attorney General Jeff Sessions is allegedly endeavoring to fortify government marijuana laws and cause states to uphold them.

Marijuana Tax Act of 1937

By 1937, the Marijuana Tax Act adequately prohibited clearance of the plant by forcing overwhelming extract charges marked down, ownership, or transportation of hemp. This demonstration, set by the U.S. government, lead to the main marijuana-related capture in October of 1937 of fiftyeight-year-old Samuel Caldwell, a rancher discovered selling cannabis.

Despite the fact that marijuana kept on being developed in the United States, the last official hemp fields were planted in Wisconsin, in 1957.

Dr. Aung-Din, Neurology and Neuro-Psychiatry expert, has for some time been an advocate of restorative cannabis for treatment of an assortment of illnesses, including epilepsy and even malignancies. Furthermore, even Dr. Aung-Din guarantees the early endeavors of the legislature during the 1900s still affect how the medication is dealt with today.

"The Marijuana Tax Act, exacted a tremendous duty with the goal that individuals would [be] prevented from purchasing cannabis. In this way, 1941, cannabis was expelled from all pharmacopeias —(you could not get it in stores and yu could not discover any proof of it). Furthermore, from that point forward, there has been disgrace and I was even dependent upon that in medicinal school" said Dr. Aung-Din to The Street.

"War on Drugs"

By 1970, the Controlled Substances Act, as a major aspect of the *War on Drugs* started by President Richard Nixon, revoked the Marijuana Tax Act, yet arranged cannabis as a Schedule 1 medication, in a similar classification as heroin, LSD, cocaine and euphoria. Medications, as indicated by the organization, were open foe number one.

Marijuana stays a Schedule 1 medication today, making extraordinary troubles for those wishing study its therapeutic properties, as Dr. Aung-Din has seen. In opposition to various therapeutic feelings, the meaning of Schedule 1 appears to conflict with marijuana's real advantages.

"A portion of my partners have confidence in the viability [of marijuana]. Yet it is possible that they cannot utilize it since they are related with colleges or emergency clinics which get government awards, so they cannot utilize it, or they are hesitant to utilize it and have the DEA coming after them since it is as yet named as a controlled substance class 1. Which implies, by definition, no therapeutic utilize and exceptionally addictive" says Dr. Aung-Din.

All things considered, Nixon's Act to a great extent overlooked the National Commission on Marijuana and Drug Abuse's report in 1972 titled *Marijuana: A Signal of Misunderstanding*, which provoked lesser punishments for little belongings and steady restriction.

Reefer Madness

The generally well known movie Reefer *Madness*, discharged in 1936, filled parental worry over marijuana utilize, and spread dread that the young people of U.S.A confronted insidious marijuana dealers that would degenerate them and lead to things like wrongdoing and sex.

In spite of the fact that culture in the end started to turn out to be increasingly instructed about the genuine impacts of cannabis use, the movie and culture encompassing it penetrated society profoundly and depicted marijuana as a passage medication to considerably progressively hazardous substances, a generalization that exists today.

In any case, with the ongoing furor over marijuana stocks and organizations, some are asserting another sort of world renowned *reefer franticness* is going on.

First Legalization of Medical Marijuana

Through the Compassionate Use Act of 1996, California formally was the primary state to authorize medicinal marijuana for use by patients with incessant diseases.

Following its example, 1990s saw the legitimization in four different States in addition to Washington D.C. for therapeutic marijuana, including Oregon, Washington, Alaska and Maine. By the mid 2000s, more States (including Nevada, Montana, Rhode Island, Hawaii, Vermont and New Mexico) passed therapeutic marijuana laws.

Since 2010, sixteen States have legitimized the medicinal utilization of marijuana.

First Legalization of Recreational Marijuana

Washington state and Vermont were the initial two states to set a ballot to legitimize the recreational utilization of marijuana, in 2012. Colorado's Proposition 64 made grown-up ownership (those more than 21 years-old) what is more business deal lawful.

A few states pursued, as of now leaving recreational marijuana lawful in nine States in addition to Washington D.C. States that have Legalized Marijuana (in some structure). From 2018 there are 30 states in addition to Washington D.C. that have legitimized marijuana in some structures. Those States are Alaska, Arkansas, Arizona, California, Colorado, Connecticut, Delaware, Washington D.C., Florida, Hawaii, Illinois, Louisiana, Maine, Maryland, Massachusetts, Michigan, Minnesota, Montana, New Hampshire, Nevada, New Jersey, New Mexico, New York, North Dakota, Ohio, Oregon, Pennsylvania, Rhode Island, Vermont, Washington and West Virginia.

First Marijuana IPO

On 2018 July 19th the main marijuana IPO in the United States (Canadian organization Tilray) started exchanging at twentythree dollars on the Nasdaq.

Since its IPO, Tilray shares have been out and out a crazy ride, with shares hitting highs of about three hundred dollars in an exchanging session prior this week.

What's Next for Marijuana?

As indicated by an examination by the Arcview Market Research and BDS Analytics, the North American marijuana advertise made an amazing 9.7 billion dollars a year ago, up 33% from the earlier year. What is more, as indicated by their appraisals, the lawful marijuana industry is anticipated to create thirty-two billion dollars of by and large worldwide monetary effect by 2022.

Moreover, one out of four youthful grown-ups utilizes marijuana, as indicated by a Gallup survey in 2018. Furthermore, with 64% of Americans supporting the sanctioning of marijuana, it appears just as government legitimization isn't excessively distant.

Enterprises and businesses the same appear to fire up for the unavoidable across the board sanctioning. Indeed Coca-Cola (KO - Get Report) as of late declared expectations to break into the cannabis business with an imbued beverage. And keeping in mind that Aurora Cannabis Inc. (ACBFF) may not be their expected accomplice, unmistakably the liquor business is hoping to gain by the huge developing business sector.

Various types of Marijuana

Marijuana has been utilized in an assortment of ways, including for therapeutic and recreational purposes. Various types of marijuana, like CBD (cannabidiol), THC and therapeutic marijuana, have been legitimized at different interims in different States in the United States.

Restorative marijuana

For a huge number of years, various societies have been utilizing marijuana for its therapeutic properties. In 1830s Irish specialist Sir William Brooke O'Shaughnessy found marijuana's advantages in treating queasiness and agony in cholera patients, in India. This lead to the across the board deal and utilization of cannabis as a solution for an assortment of stomach afflictions in Europe and even the United States (basically by specialists and drug stores in the later nineteenth century).

Today, various mixes of marijuana like CBD and THC are being utilized to treat an assortment of conditions, like epilepsy and malignant growth related diseases.

CBD (cannabidiol)

CBD is the non-psychoactive part of marijuana that is frequently connected with its medical advantages, including assuaging tension and despondency, while THC, the psychoactive segment, instigates rest or sleepiness.

Since CBD and THC do not work in a similar way (and effectsly affect the body), they have seen shifting uses throughout the years, explicitly in the medicinal field.

The first CBD-based medication, Epidiolex, by GD Pharmaceuticals (GWPH) , was endorsed prior in 2018 by the FDA, in order to treat epilepsy. Specialists trust it might trigger more extensive FDA endorsement of CBD-based medications and prescriptions. Kris Krane, leader of 4Front Ventures, considers the endorsement like a snowball impact that could divert patients from progressively hazardous other options.

"I do consider it to be a positive advancement by and large. I know there are different organizations out there that are taking a shot at various kinds of cannabinoid-based medications, so I believe it is probably going to introduce another period of cannabinoid-based pharmaceuticals and that is by and large positive" said Krane to TheStreet. He also said that *"The more passages patients need to take cannabis or cannabinoid medication, the better. Since they are successful in treating a scope of conditions, it very well may be an option in contrast to sedatives."*

THC

THC, or tetrahydrocannabinol, is the psychoactive part of marijuana and it was and and it is the most important part of debate of the plant's use.

While customary recreational utilization of the cannabis plant may have included smoking significant levels of THC for strict or different services, late hundreds of years have seen the compound changed into anything from tinctures to chewy candies and edibles.

Moreover, manufactured THC has additionally been utilized to make the medication Marinol, utilized for treating sickness and retching related with malignant growth treatment

Where did pot come from?

It is imperative to recognize the two well-known subspecies of the cannabis plant, as said by Warf. *Cannabis sativa*, known as marijuana, has psychoactive properties. The other plant is *Cannabis sativa L.* (The L was incorporated into the name to pay tribute to the botanist Carl Linnaeus.) This subspecies is known as hemp; it is a nonpsychoactive type of cannabis, and it is utilized in assembling items, for example, oil, material and fuel.

A second psychoactive types of the plant, *Cannabis indica*, was distinguished by the French naturalist Jean-Baptiste Lamarck, and a third phenomenal one, *Cannabis ruderalis*, was named in 1924 by Russian botanist D.E. Janischevisky.

Cannabis plants are accepted to have developed on the steppes of Central Asia, explicitly in the areas between Mongolia and southern Siberia, as indicated by Warf. The historical backdrop of cannabis use comes back similar to 12,000 years, which puts the plant among humankind's most seasoned developed crops, as indicated by data in the book *Marihuana: The First Twelve Thousand Years* (Springer, 1980).

"It likely prospered in the supplement rich dump destinations of ancient trackers and gatherers" wrote Warf in his investigation.

Consumed cannabis seeds have likewise been found in kurgan entombment hills in Siberia (3,000 B.C.) and a portion of the tombs of Xinjiang, in China (around 2500 B.C.) have included enormous amounts of embalmed psychoactive marijuana.

Both hemp and psychoactive marijuana were utilized broadly in old China. The primary record of the medication's restorative use dates to 4000 B.C. The herb was utilized, for example, as an analgesic during medical procedure, and stories state it was even utilized by the (genuine or legendary) Chinese Emperor Shen Nung in 2737 B.C. From China, beach front ranchers carried pot to Korea around 2000 B.C. or on the other hand prior, as per the book *The Archeology of Korea* (Cambridge University Press, 1993). Cannabis went toward the South Asian subcontinent between 2000 B.C. and 1000 B.C., when the district was attacked by the Aryans, a gathering that spoke an obsolete Indo-European language. The medication turned out to be generally utilized in India, where it was commended as one of *five realms of herbs which discharge us from tension* in one of the antiquated Sanskrit Vedic ballads whose name convert into *Study of Charms*.

From Asia to Europe

Cannabis went to the Middle East between 2000 B.C. and 1400 B.C., and it was presumably utilized there by the Scythians, a migrant Indo-European gathering. The Scythians additionally likely conveyed the medication into southeast of Russia and Ukraine, as they involved the two domains for a considerable length of time, as indicated by Warf's report. Germanic clans brought the medication into Germany, and marijuana went from that point to Britain during the 5th century with the Anglo-Saxon intrusions.

"Cannabis seeds have additionally been found in the remaining parts of Viking ships dating to the mid-ninth century" Warf wrote in the examination.

Throughout the following hundreds of years, cannabis moved to different districts of the world, going through Africa, arriving in South America in the 19th century, then arriving in North America.

How Did Marijuana Get To The United States?

After this truly long *trip* all through the pre-present day and current universes, cannabis at long last went to the United States toward the start of the 20th century. It landed in the southwest of United States from Mexico, with foreigners escaping that Nation during the Mexican Revolution of 1910-1911.

"Numerous early partialities against marijuana were not at all subtle bigot fears of its smokers, regularly proclaimed by reactionary papers" wrote Warf in his report. He also added: *"Mexicans were as often as possible accused for smoking marijuana, property violations, enticing kids and taking part in dangerous binges."*

26

Americans laws never perceived the distinction between *Cannabis sativa L.* and *Cannabis sativa.* The plant was first banned in Utah in 1915, and by 1931 it was illicit in 29 states, as indicated by the report.

In 1930, Harry Aslinger turned into the main official of the Federal Bureau of Narcotics (FBN) and attempted numerous endeavors to make marijuana illicit in all states. In 1937, the Marijuana Tax Act put cannabis under the guideline of the Drug Enforcement Agency, condemning ownership of the plant all through the nation.

"Today, the government still characterizes marijuana as a Schedule controlled substance, alongside heroin and LSD, showing it has high potential for misuse and habit, no acknowledged medicinal uses and no sheltered degree of utilization" said Warf.

PHASES OF THE MARIJUANA PLANT LIFE CYCLE

Is it true you are interested about the regular life cycle of the cannabis plant? Would you like to take a stab at delivering your own marijuana reap but are you uncertain about how, precisely, to go about it? Well have we got a treat for you.

In this book the specialists at Honest Marijuana will inspect the seven key phases of the marijuana plant life cycle. En route, we will talk about:

- The significance of marking the sex of your seeds

- How to support germination

- How to perceive embryonic leaves on a marijuana plant seedling

- The significance of light during the vegetative stage

- The distinction between the male and female plants

- Why you have to disconnect the female plants on the off chance that you need to deliver the most bud

- The most ideal approaches to collect and safeguard your marijuana plant

- Planning for the following developing season

From that point forward, we will control you through the whole development procedure of the marijuana plant, from germination to seedling. Through vegetation, pre-flowering, and flowering; to collecting and the following seed life-cycle phases of your pot plant.

So, lash yourself in for a wild ride through the essential science of your preferred weed. It is certain to be a pleasant outing. We will begin our adventure where every single great voyages start: at the cause, the source, the seed.

STAGE 1: THE MARIJUANA PLANT SEED

Get any seed and inspect it intently. Turn it over and around. Feel the weight. Notice the shape and the shading. Presently let me know whether that seed is going to deliver a male marijuana plant or a female marijuana plant. Cannot do it, can you? Try not to feel terrible. Nobody can do it.

In any case, that brings a significant issue into the universe of do-it-without anyone's help ganja developing: how might you be certain the seeds you plant will deliver the marijuana you need? This is a significant inquiry on the grounds that solitary the female plant delivers the trichome-rich cola buds that you can collect to smoke, vape, touch and ingest.

The male plant creates none of that. Indeed, the male marijuana plant can really be a burden to your cannabis collect, whenever become together with female plants. This is on the grounds that the male plant's sole design is to fertilize the female plants. And keeping in mind that does not seem like an awful thing: it really is.

At the point when female marijuana plants are pollinated, they start utilizing their vitality to create seeds and quit utilizing their vitality to sustain the buds that we as a whole know and love. Enabling a male plant to develop close by a female plant is a formula for decreased bud reap, and it can demolish the euphoric properties of the female cannabis plant's high-prompting *organic product*. Be certain you separate all male and female plants immediately.

So, as should be obvious, it is great to know whether your ganja seeds will deliver female plants or male plants before you start developing them. Be that as it may, that takes us back to the previous inquiry: how might you be certain the seeds you plant will deliver the marijuana you need?

Numerous marijuana seeds can resemble the other the same along these lines. So, the best way to know without a doubt if the seed you are holding is male or female is to name it, following expelling it from the plant. Presently, clearly, you cannot name the seed itself, however you can place the seeds in a compartment with different seeds of a similar sex.

In the model photograph underneath, you can see the minor seed in what appears to be a shot glass or little candleholder. The paper mark on the front shows the strain (Skunk Special) and the sex (F for female) of this specific seed.

Also, just to be clear, you do not have to store every individual seed in its own holder. You can fill the holder with seeds as long as they are no different strain and no different sex. Just figured we should express that inside and out before you blow all your well-deserved assets on a gazillion little compartments.

For those of you on a financial limit, the least complex holder is a paper sack or envelope. However also different sorts will work. Simply ensure that you do not store your seeds in a plastic sack or some other hermetically sealed compartment. The dampness that gets caught inside will make the seed form and become futile.

Whatever holder you pick, make certain to check it with the strain name and the sex of the plant, so you can keep your strains isolated.

At the point when you are done arranging your seeds, it is an ideal opportunity to proceed onward to the following stage in the marijuana plant life cycle.

STAGE 2: GERMINATION

Germination is the improvement of a plant from a seed or spore after a time of torpidity. When you expel the seed from the marijuana plant, it will go lethargic until it is presented to dampness. That implies that on the off chance that you keep the seeds dry, you can store them for as long as a year without influencing, practicality.

Would it be advisable for you to grow both the male and female seeds so as to deliver quality buds for recreational or therapeutic use? We will respond to that question in the following two areas.

Separate The Males

Now, you ought to have a heap of male seeds to your left side and a heap of female seeds to your right side. The side each sex is on does not generally make a difference insofar as they are isolated. In the case that you need male seeds on the privilege and female seeds on the left, more capacity to you.

Presently get together the male seeds and store them in a dim, dry wardrobe or cabinet. Actually, put them in a completely unique room as a sanity check. You are not going to require them, and you would prefer not to take any risk that they will some way or another influence your female plants.

There truly is no danger of cross-sullying except if you plant the male seeds and enable them to develop and develop. We were simply waxing hyperbolic in the past passage to underscore exactly how irrelevant the male seeds are.

Develop The Females

Presently take the female seeds and absorb them some water or crease them up in a soggy paper towel. There could be odds you have either done the moist paper towel test in science class or you know somebody who did. So it should not be an unexpected that you can begin the developing procedure with simply a touch of dampness.

On the off chance that you pick some water choice, you may see that a few seeds will coast from the outset. Try not to stress. They will in the long run sink to the base as they ingest water, become soaked, and grow.

Remember that a solitary marijuana plant can develop to five feet tall with a wingspan (separation left to right) of a few feet. That can top off a room rather rapidly. The key moment that arranging your develop is to give each plant a lot of room. Try not to grow 20 seeds except if you have the area to oblige that much organic issue.

Leave the wet seed canvassed in a warm dim spot for twenty-four hours until the seed grows its taproot. At the point when the taproot rises, expel the seed from some water or the sodden paper towel and plant it in some great, sound earth or topsoil.

The taproot will at that point connect itself to the topsoil and start absorbing the supplements it needs to proceed in the development cycle. In the end, the seed will drive another stem up past the outside of the topsoil. In this manner starts the seedling phase of the marijuana plant life cycle.

STAGE 3: SEEDLING

During the seedling stage, two embryonic leaves will open outward from the stem to get the daylight that the little plant needs to break out of its underground seed packaging. The embryonic leaves will look not at all like the marijuana leaves that you are utilized.

The following pair of leaves to develop from the young plant will be the first to have the exemplary adjusted focuses that make the marijuana leaf stand apart from all the rest. The marijuana leaf is unmistakable to such an extent that numerous individuals, in the cannabis network, use it as an image to speak to their way of life.

With everything taken into account, the seedling will develop somewhere in the range of four and eight leaves during this phase of its improvement. The seedling stage can last somewhere in the range of one to three weeks relying upon:

- Soil type

- Strain of marijuana developed

- Amount of water the seed gets

- Airflow

- Humidity

- Duration of light

- Quality of light

In the case this is your first or second develop (or even your third, fourth, or fiftieth), you should concentrate on growing a sound plant instead of the precise measure of time it takes to overcome each stage. We simply supply these general numbers to give you a thought of what to look for your plant develops.

So do not blow a gasket if the seedling stage is a day or two short of a week or stretches somewhat over three weeks. It is only a plant. Truly, the final product is your own one of a kind homegrown ganja, yet it is not worth getting worked up about. You can generally go purchase a baggie of your preferred strain from your close dispensary.

That gets us to the following stage the life of the marijuana plant: the vegetative (or vegetation) stage.

STAGE 4: VEGETATION STAGE

During the vegetation stage, the stem will become thicker and taller and they will start to grow new hubs. These hubs will create more leaves and even new branches.

Since it is developing and creating leaves and branches, your plant will require a lot of crisp warm water alongside:

•   Flowing, dry air

•   Lots of nitrogen-rich natural supplements (e.g., fluid fish or seaweed)

•   As much soil space as could be expected under the circumstances

The entirety of this together permits your marijuana plant to develop from an eight-inch young plant into an a few foot tall tree inside the range of three to about a month and a half.

The development of the plant to a great extent relies upon the rate its leaves can accumulate daylight and change it into concoction vitality (photosynthesis). This reality clarifies why the vegetative plant will require extended periods of summer daylight (from twelve to, at least, fifteen in the wild) or eighteen hours of bright light every day.

The THC tree will stop its upward development once it begins getting less regular outdoor sunlight or when the indoor cultivator diminishes the plant from eighteen to twelve hours of glaring light every day. It is now that the plant enters the pre-flowering stage.

It can take somewhere in the range of one to five months for the developing marijuana plant to enter the pre-flowering stage. At the point you will have the option to confirm that you did for sure plant all females.

On the off chance that the plant is a male, you will see minimal green banana-like sack structures on the hub locales of the plant, where the leaves meet the principle stem. These sack structures hold dust and they will just show up on male plants. Male plants must be isolated from female plants before the little green sacs burst open and discharge their dust. In the case that you do not locate the male plants in time, and the sacs do blast, the dust can treat the cola of the close by female plants. This fertilization ruins the psychoactive capability of the trichomes the female plant may develop.

At the point when you keep your female marijuana plant from being pollinated by a male plant, you produce what is known as a *sinsemilla*. Sinsemilla (in English *without seed*) alludes to a female marijuana plant that does not have any seeds since it has not been treated by dust. Sinsemilla plants produce a lot of tar just as phony seedpods, the two of which contain high rates of THC.

You can recognize sinsemilla plants by the white hairs that rise up out of the pear-molded bracts at their plant hubs. Remember that occasionally, a plant can be bisexual. This implies it has the two arrangements of regenerative (organs and leaves).

Bisexual cannabis plants can really fertilize themselves and ruin your THC or CBD collect. Thus, it is imperative to stay careful and to isolate and devastate any androgynous plants with female organs and male leaves that convey the possibility to fertilize and destroy your psychoactive sinsemilla.

When the light term starts to diminish (regardless of whether normally or falsely), the cannabis plant moves into the flowering stage. That is the place we will go straightaway.

STAGE 6: FLOWERING

Your plant will keep on developing into sticks and leaves without creating any of the bloom's therapeutic characteristics, except if its light presentation is step by step diminished. This may mean less time spent in the sunlight or by misleadingly diminishing indoor glaring light time from eighteen to twelve hours.

During the flowering stage, your pot plant will likewise require potassium and phosphorus-based supplements, for example, bat guano, so as to set blossoms appropriately. At the point when it does, however, you will start to see and smell moist trichome-soaked cola buds developing from your plant.

These buds will likewise deliver long, flimsy, smooth white hairs, or pistils, that will start to rise throughout the following eight to ten weeks. The entirety of this flowering movement is activated by a straightforward decrease in light.

You will realize your cannabis plant is ready for reap when the shades of the pistils on the cola buds change from smooth white to ruddy orange. You will likewise need to utilize a magnifying instrument to check the shade of the leaders of the trichomes overflowing out from the ready cola buds.

You will realize that your buds are prepared for reap when the trichome heads abandon clear to smooth and dark to golden. The nearness of increasingly golden trichome heads will probably demonstrate a higher CBD to THC cannabinoid profile proportion in its trichome gum.

On the off chance that you need to gather your marijuana plant for its full THC or CBD impacts, you DO NOT need the trichomes to tumble off. On the off chance that that occurs, that implies that you let the plant become excessively long. Most of the cannabinoids are presently gone, you won't appreciate the psychoactive or therapeutic impacts, and you will need to begin growing another group of marijuana.

Rather, numerous cultivators recommend collecting the crop when a large portion of the trichomes on the plant are dark. In principle, this creates the most elevated level of THC with the least degree of CBD (which neutralizes the euphoric impacts of the previous).

The little hairs that develop from inside the calyxes or the pistils are another hint that encourages you decide when to collect your cannabis, for the particular sort of substance properties you need it to contain. The shade of the pistils changes from brilliant white to corroded orange or darker toward the finish of the plant's flowering stage.

Toward one side of the range, on the off chance that you see a higher proportion of white to red guns, that implies your pot will deliver to a greater extent an euphoric THC high. On the opposite finish of the range, in the event that you see a higher proportion of red to white guns, that implies your pot will deliver to a greater extent a calm, quiet CBD stoned inclination.

Soundly in the middle of those two boundaries, cannabis crops gathered in the flowering cycle, when generally a large portion of the trichome heads are murky and the pistils are not yet darker, should deliver an increasingly adjusted THC-to-CBD mix of cannabinoids.

At the point when you have established that it is without a doubt time to gather your bud, you will need a decent pair of scissors or a sharp pruning device to cut the storage compartment from the roots so it very well may be dried.

Make the slice as near the base of the plant as could be allowed. At that point continue to cut the tree into littler branches. Doing so will make it simpler to dry the plant.

When you have cut your plant into little segments, string up the pieces and hang them topsy turvy from lines of twine in a dim, cool live with a moistness level of forty to fifty percent. The plant matter ought to remain hanging along these lines and in these conditions for four to six days.

While you are cutting your pot plant into segments for drying, trim the leaves and stems and put them in a safe spot. This material can be cut away, spared, and in the long run prepared to make cannabutter and cannabis concentrate after your buds have dried.

When your buds are finished drying, place them in a wide-mouthed glass bricklayer container with a screw top. Fill the containers to simply underneath the top and do not pack the buds in. Doing so will diminish wind current and cause issues later on. Store the artisan shakes in a storage room where the temperature remains somewhere in the range of fifty and sixty Fahrenheit degrees.

Your containers ought to stay here for one to three weeks, so, as to fix the buds and finish the collecting procedure. When daily you have to air out the containers. This enables natural air to get in and any gases delivered by the relieving procedure to get out.

MEDICAL MARIJUANA GROWING GUIDE

Medicinal marijuana is legitimate in right around fourteen states in the US and this is because of the way that specialists accept that marijuana has recuperating properties. Under the government law, developing marijuana, utilizing it or having it in your ownership is a criminal offense and it is significant that except if you have your doctor's suggestion to utilize it, you do not consider developing this substance at home.

How do I get the seeds?

The speediest and maybe the most immediate approach to get your hands on certain seeds is get them from somebody who as of now has their very own develop arrangement (Legitimately, an individual can offer up to an ounce in seeds, like the law encompassing gifting gathered marijuana. You can likewise have up to ten ounces of marijuana in your home, albeit any sum over an ounce must be bolted up).

In any case, on the off chance that you do not have that alternative, you might have the option to discover some somewhere else.

State guidelines take into account authorized retailers to sell seeds, however it is not clear as of right now if dispensaries will have those in stock.

Numerous individuals buy seeds on the web, in spite of the fact that it is critical to take note of that under government law, both having marijuana (seeds included) and mailing it crosswise over state lines stays unlawful.

Web based shopping can likewise be somewhat hazardous, as indicated by Will Ried, supervisor of Rootdown Hydroponics Indoor Garden Center in Medford, who alerts that in case you are getting seeds from an arbitrary dealer, you may not be getting your cash's value.

By and large, seed costs change. A gander of a couple of online merchants demonstrated costs somewhere in the range of 20 dollars and 200 dollars, contingent upon the strain and what number of seeds you need (what number are in a solitary pack additionally shifts, between retailers).

For individuals who have gotten a permit to develop marijuana lawfully, it is significant that you become familiar with the procedures of developing and developing marijuana. Given beneath is a short restorative marijuana developing guide that can assist you with understanding the procedure better.

1. Seeds Customary cannabis plants are either male or female.

On the off chance that you buy standard seeds, each seed in this way has a fifty-fifty possibility of developing into that one. Male plants are useful in case you are hoping to create more seeds, however female plants, which have greater blossoms with higher cannabinoid levels, are the ones you will need to collect, as indicated by Matt Reisman, proprietor of Gardin Hydroponics and Soil in Braintree. It can make a parcel of standard seeds a genuine test and a genuine bet.

For apprentices, Reisman prescribes developing from feminized seeds. Seeds that, to put it plainly, are made to not make any male plants.

2. Picking a space to develop

Some incredible spots incorporate storm cellars, storage rooms and upper rooms. Regardless of which indoor area you pick, ensure that it approaches electrical outlets.

3. Holders

You should develop your plant in a pot or a compartment. Continuously ensure that you utilize enormous plastic pots.

4. Temperature and lighting

As a rule, marijuana plants require around eighty degrees during the day and around fifty degrees around evening time.

Eighteen hours of light is required for customary cannabis seeds to develop in the vegetative cycle. To bloom, the plants ought to have an even twelve-hour split between red-orange light and murkiness.

In the event that you develop the plant indoors, at that point there are no chances for your plant to get adequate daylight. Since plants like marijuana need a ton of daylight to develop well, you can utilize fake lighting to give your plant all the light it needs to develop. Some incredible alternatives incorporate glaring lights, metal halide lights and high pressure sodium lights.

5. Consider the components that will influence the photosynthesis

Aside from the measure of light arriving at the plants, there are different elements that will influence the pace of photosynthesis. These incorporate stickiness, temperature, carbon dioxide, water, and so forth.

6. What extent does it take to develop?

The developing procedure fluctuates long, however it ordinarily takes at any rate four-and-a-half months for a little develop.

Be that as it may, auto-flowering plants, which originate from an alternate strain, as per Leafly, require just from seventy to seventy-five days to develop and blossom and

they do not need bother with any adjustments in their lighting period, said Dan Ruta, director of Gardin Hydroponics and Soil.

The tradeoff for the quicker procedure however is that these little plants produce less to reap, he said.

7. What amount of marijuana would I be able to collect from one plant?

There is no basic answer. Numerous components play into what you end up with, including the strain, to what extent you let the plant vegetate, and what sort of supplements you use. *"There is an extremely considerable rundown of factors that apply to a yield"* What is sure, in any case, is that you will need to re-seed each year, he said. Cannabis is certifiably not a perpetual plant.

8. Collecting

The best time to collect begins when the plants flowering. Trust that the flowering procedure will finish. Cut the plants, expel the lower huge leaves and spot the plants in shoe boxes. Mix them around every day as this will assist them with drying rapidly. When the plants have dried totally, they are prepared for use.

Our association with cannabis apparently starts and finishes with development. All types of cannabis that we devour get from a developed plant. The estimation of the cannabis plant, restorative or something else, is to a great extent subject to what we do with it, how and when we develop it, how we refine it for our own utilization and even what words we use to portray it.

Cannabis is a dioecious plant, meaning it tends to be categorically isolated into male and female plants. Male plants produce the dust important for a female plant to deliver seeds, while the female plant is the one to naturally create a greater amount of the major cannabinoids, specifically cannabidiolic corrosive (CBDA) and tetrahydrocannabinolic corrosive (THCA), which convert to CBD and THC, separately. Cannabis additionally delivers a few other important mixes, for example, terpenes and flavonoids, that potentially work synergistically with the cannabinoids to improve wanted and remedial impacts.

While still profoundly discussed, most nations just remember one cannabis animal categories, *Cannabis sativa L.*, yet some perceive up to three species: C. sativa, C. indica, and C. ruderalis, in light of geographic origin, hereditary qualities, and morphology. The focal contrast between the present indica and sativa plants is in their perceptible attributes during the development cycle.

Indica plants will in general develop short with thick stems and expansive, dark green leaves. They additionally have shorter flowering cycles, and develop adequately in chilly, short-season atmospheres. Sativa plants have longer flowering cycles, toll better in warm atmospheres with long seasons, and usually become taller with moderately light-green and restricted leaves.

Knowing the morphological or physical structure contrasts among indica and sativa plants is more helpful to producers and cultivators than virtually any other individual in the cannabis space, in spite of the terms' normal use in the purchaser commercial center.

Cannabis has been reproduced by people for three distinct purposes:

Fiber – harvesting cannabis stalks, typically from hemp assortments.

Seeds – harvesting seeds from a female hemp plant for its rich oil and protein content.

Medication type cultivars — harvesting developed assortments for their psychoactive and remedial cannabinoids.

From seed to gather, the cannabis plant's development cycle can last somewhere in the range of ten to twenty-six weeks. The cycle has three main stages: germination, vegetation, and flowering. Like most plants, cannabis requires light, air, supplements, and a medium to house its underlying foundations. The sum and length of light the plant is presented to directs which development organize it will be in.

Nearby Cannabis Cultivation Laws and Regulations

In many nations and nearby wards where cannabis is lawful (medically or recreationally) some kind of home growing is typically allowed, however growing laws change altogether from nation to nation and even from city to city. In case you are an imminent or current home cultivator, you should know the laws and guidelines of your ward.

Cannabis Plant Sex and Anatomy

Male and female cannabis plants share a typical fundamental life systems of roots, stems, and leaves. Both plant genders produce trichomes, the glandular members on the outside of the bloom, which create and hold the plant's cannabinoids and terpenes, be that as it may, the female plant delivers unquestionably more trichomes than the male plant. Past these nuts and bolts, cannabis life structures shifts essentially among male and female plants.

The Cannabis Farmer's Guide To Water-Absorbent Polymers

Probably the greatest challenge an outdoor cannabis cultivator can be defied with are drawn out times of super hot, dry climate. Each ganja rancher fears dry spell. Water-retentive polymers are a lifeline and you really can dry spell evidence your plantation on the off chance that you continue reading Innovative work by the United States Department of Agriculture (USDA), during the 1960s prompted the making of the primary hydrogel model AKA Super Slurper. Early items that pursued were granulated sugar-like powders, tiny plastic gems that looked like slime when wet. Continued private innovative work have driven us to biodegradable precious stones with huge water retention limit.

Water-retentive polymers, superabsorbent polymers, and hydrogels are very similar. In any case, the best present day, durable, agriculture grade polymers can hold thierty–sixty their own volume of wate, without leaving behind any poisonous side-effects in the topsoil.

Polyacrylate polymers are usually sodium-based. They can be regularly found in diapers/nappies. The issue begins with PACs after around a half year as they begin to separate. Not exclusively is this most likely too early for plants, limiting the quantity of wet/dry cycles, and it is additionally a potential collect spoiler. These polymers discharge nitrogen even under the least favorable conditions, typically when most photoperiod strains are in late blossom. Or on the other hand more regrettable, during flushing.

Conversely, potassium-based polyacrylamides (PAMs) take five–seven years to weaken. Today, many are biodegradable. You can develop any strain you like again and again. PAMs can enable a cultivator to preserve water and composts long haul. The best part is that these polymers are genuinely environmentally neighborly. Ensured not to defer or taint your reap.

Auto cultivators can likely pull off using the precious stones cut from packs of diapers. Given that most autoflowering half and halves have a total lifecycle of somewhere close to eight–twelve weeks. Remember. time is your ally. So you do not really require polymers with a long lifespan. Entirely conventional develop hack for one auto crop.

Be that as it may, on the off chance that you intend to develop outdoors for a half year or more, the development of some photoperiod beast plants requests more excellent polymers. You need superabsorbent gel or powder that can maintain powerful wet/dry cycles for a time of years, as opposed to months. Alsta Hydrogel by Chemtex Speciality Limited is a great eco-accommodating choice.

A cup loaded with superabsorbent precious stones goes far. The best method to utilize hydrogel is to hydrate it first. Ideally with a light supplement arrangement. At that point, blend the jam in with the base third of soil in an enormous container or profound opening. On the other hand, Just a couple of grams of dry powder should be added to the dirt blend. See the maker's guidelines on the document or visit their site for particulars.

Essentially, you are creating a crisis repository for the plant's, underlying foundations to take advantage of when they need it most. On the off chance that you expect delayed dry spell conditions, you can blend polymers all through the dirt network to improve the overall water maintenance properties of the substrate of the topsoil. The special reward is a superior circulated air through medium and progressively proficient utilization of composts.

Only one out of every odd outdoor crop is a level green field with columns of cannabis plants. A lot of guerrilla cultivators are cultivating marijuana on sloping slopes. The mystery is they are using hydrogel to lessen water overflow. Likewise, hydrogel proves to be useful on the off chance that you do not have the advantage of planting near and dear and cannot make day by day outings to water plants. During the most driest summer months, polymer stores can keep plants from drying out and wilting for a day or two longer.

We have seen some promising outcomes with another kind of supplement film system (NFT, for example, hydrogel film that has been utilized to develop some fabulous hydroponic lettuce in Japan. Sadly, this new develop tech has battled to deliver abundant harvests of bigger fruiting plant species. Until further notice, water-retentive polymers are only soil enhancers.

All-In-1 GrowCaps are an outstanding case of how polymers can improve cannabis growing. These GrowCaps highlight capsuled polymers that gradually discharge supplements after some time. They contain all of the supplements that cannabis plants require over the whole develop cycle, however they do not dump it into the dirt all immediately.

The polymers gradually separate over the regular development cycle, meaning the right supplements are constantly accessible in the ideal amounts. In such manner, polymers have made growing cannabis more available than any other time in recent memory. Tenderfoots need not stress over juggling supplement proportions and feeding plans. It is only a matter of placing GrowCaps in the dirt and watching the enchantment unfurl.

All-In-1 GrowCaps don't simply make feeding simpler, they additionally diminish water utilization by 30%. They assimilate water with incredible proficiency and discharge it once more into the dirt gradually after some time.

Through the span of our common history with cannabis, creators, researchers, producers, and industry insiders have utilized competing terms to portray the equivalent conceptive plant anatomy. Because of a broad time of restriction, herbal terms have been every now and again abused or supplanted totally. Likewise, mainstream conversational terms have gotten interchangeable regardless of having various meanings

Thus, how about we alleviate a portion of the disarray and guide out the anatomy of both plant genders by first identifying organic terms, at that point clearing up a portion of the regular idioms we have inherited.

ANATOMY OF THE FEMALE PLANT

The female cannabis plant is a pistillate, meaning it has pistils and marks of disgrace. You may have heard female cannabis plants alluded to as *sinsemilla*, deciphered from Spanish as *without seeds*. Sensemilla alludes to all non-pollinated female plants. Sensemilla plants are perfect for marijuana cultivators since they offer the most elevated potential yield of cannabinoids. Pollinated female blooms, or female blossoms with seeds, produce a less attractive item than blooms from seedless marijuana.

The regenerative anatomy of the female plant includes:

Colas: The blossoms delivered by the female plant. Colas are secured with cannabinoid-and terpene-rich trichomes and normally called buds or nugs. A cannabis bud is not to be mistaken for the natural definition of the word bud: a recently emerging plant.

Bracts: Small, scale-like leaf structures that embody and ensure the seeds. Bracts are regularly alluded to as calyxes, however this term is botanically incorrect. The female cannabis plant does, in any case, have calyx cells within the sensitive layer of tissue between the seed and the bracts that exemplify it.

Marks of shame: The regenerative pieces of the cannabis plant, which gets dust from the male plant. Marks of disgrace are ordinarily and incorrectly alluded to as pistils. Two marks of shame project from one pistil.

Pistil: The regenerative pieces of the female cannabis bloom that are enacted if dust is caught by the marks of disgrace.

Sugar Leaves: The small leaves that hold cannabis buds together. They are called sugar leaves because of the high convergence of trichomes that have a sugarlike appearance.

ANATOMY OF THE MALE PLANT

The male cannabis plant is a staminate, meaning it has stamen or dust producing regenerative organs. Male plants are some of the time developed for fiber and are all the more regularly utilized for breeding new assortments of intoxicating cannabis. During their flowering stage, male cannabis plants discharge dust, which will provoke a female plant to begin producing seeds. This training redirects vitality from blossom generation and decreases the overall yield. To augment your blossom yield and counteract seed generation, keep male and female plants isolated.

The male cannabis plant is equipped for producing cannabinoids, yet its trichomes are meagerly scattered over its surface. Guys do not create such huge numbers of trichomes as a female.

The conceptive anatomy of the male plant includes:

Stamen: The organ of the male plant that produces dust and discharges it into the wind, where it might be conveyed to the disgrace of a female plant for pollination.

Anther: The sacks that deliver and hold dust within the stamen. Anthers hang by a small fiber. Together, the anther and the fiber make up a stamen.

Dust: Microscopic grains created and contained in the anther that prepare the female plant when discharged.

BISEXUAL

A bisexual is an uncommon monecious plant, meaning it creates both male and female sex organs. The term monecious stems from the root *mono*, meaning *one*. While there are various reasons that a plant may show the two signs, bisexuals are essentially shaped if a female plant is presented to outrageous conditions during key phases of development, for example, insufficient light or unforgiving ecological conditions. Indications of a bisexual typically show late into flowering.

In a final endeavor to continue their seed line, a sensemilla crop will occasionally deliver a couple of bisexuals. While the dust of these bisexuals is much of the time unviable, marijuana cultivators should evacuate bisexuals when they jump out at eliminate the danger of pollination. Bisexuals will likewise deliver a lower overall blossom yield as the plant is compelled to redirect vitality into the creation of seeds that would have generally been utilized for the generation of trichome-rich blooms.

CANNABIS PROPAGATION TECHNIQUES

Spread incorporates the whole development cycle from begin to reap. Cannabis can be developed either from seeds or a cutting (clone) from another plant.

- **Seed**

Cannabis seeds, framed when dust prepares the female plant, are prepared to plant and develop when they effectively germinate, or once the root has gotten through the seed. While you can plant your seeds straightforwardly into the ground, it is prescribed to germinate them in a soggy paper towel before planting. Home cultivators frequently start with feminized seeds to guarantee that the grown-up plant is a flowering female.

Propagation through seeds is usually known as sexual propagation, and is a frequently favored technique for outdoor cannabis development since it makes for a progressively strong plant. Not exclusively do sexually engendered crops have a more prominent yield potential than clones, they are likewise progressively impervious to nuisances, ailments, and sicknesses.

The most often refered to disservice of growing plants from seeds is inconsistency. Plants spread by seeds do not maintain the accurate phenotype, or noticeable physical qualities and compound characteristics, of the parent plant. This causes changes and inconsistencies in the cannabinoids and terpenes that producers and customers may find unfortunate.

While a lot of cultivators need uniform plants, occasionally cultivators will grow a lot of plants from seeds so they can pick plants that produce one of a kind physical and sweet-smelling attributes. This training is regularly alluded to as pheno hunting and is drilled by most nurseries.

- **Clones**

Asexual propagation, otherwise called cloning, is the replication of a single parent plant outside the methods for sexual reproduction. Cannabis clones typically start with a cutting of a steady mother plant, which is probably going to develop into a genetically comparable plant under the correct development conditions. A clone's focal reason for existing is to replicate and save the hereditary character of a cannabis plant. At the point, when become under precisely the same ecological conditions as the mother plant, a clone is infinitely almost certain than a plant developed from seed to display the mother plant's physical attributes, just as its cannabinoid and terpene profile. It ought to likewise reflect the mother's capacity to take in supplements and oppose bugs or growths.

Since they are not presented to the hereditary qualities of different plants (instead receiving a similar hereditary code as the mother plant), clones stand a far superior possibility of preserving the ideal attributes of the mother. Plants developed from clones likewise allow producers to determine which natural conditions will maintain those perfect hereditary qualities, and determine ideal feeding plans, flowering occasions, and supplement plans.

Absence of hereditary assorted variety is something beneficial for cultivators, yet it can likewise have calamitous results. In the event that plants are presented to unfriendly ecological conditions for which they have no hereditary safeguard, a whole crop can be cleared out.

Selecting a Cannabis Growing Medium

Regardless of whether a plant is developed from a clone or seed, it needs a medium to fill in as a base for a restorative life. A growing medium is the material where plants are set during the development cycle. Regardless of whether you use hydroponics, aeroponics, or customary soil development, your chose growing medium needs to furnish the plant's underlying foundations with air, water, and supplements.

Soil

Soil is the most well-known mode for growing cannabis. Empowering soil is an exceptionally steady growing medium, allowing for adequate dampness maintenance that gives the producer abundant time between watering sessions. Soil is promptly accessible and generally simple to work with, which makes it a viable growing mode for the largest range of producers, from forthcoming home cultivators to true blue specialists. Soil can be utilized for both indoor and outdoor growing.

Hydroponics

Hydroponic development is the favored vehicle for indoor cultivators, feeding plants through a supplement rich fluid arrangement. Perlite, vermiculite, coco coir, and hydroton balls are all generally utilized hydroponic media, which allow for ideal take-up of supplements and diminished water utilization contrasted and soil. Hydroponic strategies are likewise as often as possible utilized in greenhouse settings, yet not generally utilized for outdoor growing.

The significant drawback of hydroponics is the thorough tender loving care the training requires. Hydroponic media are considerably more delicate to serious temperatures. A lot of warmth, specifically, can be very damaging as it invites microscopic organisms and malady. In the mean time, the water's pH and supplement levels must be reliably checked to guarantee the plant is getting what it needs to become solid.

Aeroponics

Aeroponics work comparatively to hydroponics, but instead than maintaining the plant's underlying foundations submerged in water, an aeroponic framework suspends the plant's foundations in a situation of fog and air where they ingest water, supplements, and oxygen. An aeroponic framework apparently has the most potential for greatest yield, but at the same time it is substantially more touchy than different frameworks. Both natural and development control factors must get cautious, steady consideration for an aeroponic framework to be successful.

Germinating Seeds or Rooting Cannabis Clones

The germination stage happens from the minute a seed's developing life is presented to water until the seed has grown its plumule, or initial taproot. Germination possibly happens when plants are developed from a seed, and usually takes between twelve hours and three weeks, depending on the essentialness of the seed, age of the seed, and germination methods chose by the producer.

The least difficult approach to germinate a cannabis seed is by placing it around three millimeters somewhere down in wet topsoil. Germination soils are likewise an alternative, structured with micronutrient mixes that encourage sound sprouting. Numerous cultivators incline toward towel germination, in which seeds are put between two moist paper towels, at that point quickly moved into a growing medium once the taproot is uncovered.

In the event that grew from a clone, the rooting stage is the time wherein the plant builds up its taproot. During this time, the youthful cutting is presented to twenty-four hours of light in a situation with high mugginess. This can take somewhere in the range of three to fourteen days.

The vegetative stage is the point at which the plant develops its underlying foundations, stalks, and enormous fan leaves that will structure the plant. Fan leaves will at last be utilized to change over the daylight into the sugars that the plant needs to deliver the blossoms or seeds. The light cycle is typically diminished to eighteen hours of light, as it requires a minimum of sixteen hours of light to maintain the plant. During cannabis vegetation, cultivators can train their plants or control their development designs for a large number of reasons. Indoor cultivators might need to train their plants to remain short by growing horizontally, while indoor and outdoor producers might need to drive their plant to build up different bloom development destinations at a similar level.

Training Techniques

There are a few training systems indoor producers send to get an ideal yield out of their plants within restricted space and lighting conditions. All of them involve manipulating the shape and development of the plant, usually by bending the stem in some style or another.

Ocean of Green (SOG)

The Sea of Green (SOG) procedure involves growing a few small plants instead of a couple of enormous ones with the intention of maximizing space and cultivating single colas. With the best possible arrangement, a SOG develop advances the most limited vegetative stage to deliver short and thick colas.

Low Stress Training (LST)

Low Stress Training (LST), like most training strategies, involves bending and tying down stems for greatest yield and light introduction within a finite space. The *low pressure* component of LST alludes to manipulating stem development for outrageous bending to anticipate the pressure that outcomes from breakage or cutting.

Super Cropping

You may think of super cropping as something contrary to LST in that it includes strategically executed types of *high pressure*, as opposed to sustained types of minimal pressure. This strategy utilizes focused on worry to urge cannabis plants to create a greater amount of the cannabinoids and terpenes they produce for insurance.

Strategically arranged and executed weight on the plant is intended to initiate a cautious response, along these lines increasing the plant's cannabinoid and terpene generation. This sort of sustained pressure is usually accomplished by pinching focused on territories of the stems and tying them down. At the point when cultivators accidentally apply an excess of stress, they typically apply channel tape to the harmed territory to enable the plant to mend.

Screen of Green (SCROG)

The Screen of Green (SCROG) strategy utilizes LST or Super Cropping to inhibit vertical development of the cannabis plant by encouraging level development. This is finished by forcing the plants to develop through a suspended even screen. As the crop stems spread laterally over the screen, colas structure in generally lethargic zones of the stem. This method is utilized where nearby laws limit the measure of plants that can be developed at one given point, allowing cultivators to utilize a bigger measure of zone.

Lollipopping

Lollipopping is removing development from the lower part of the plant to occupy vitality to the higher branches that produce colas, resulting in a *candy-* formed plant. This method is especially helpful for indoor arrangements that offer minimal light to bring down branches and regularly utilized on SCROG develops.

Topping and Fimming (FIM)

Topping comprises of clipping the growing tip of a plant's main stem at a fourty-five degree edge that makes two colas structure instead of one. This technique is utilized to keep the plant from growing like a Christmas tree by stopping the vertical development of the main stalk and allowing the lower development tips a chance to make up for lost time. Producers can likewise *top* a plant on numerous occasions to transform two development tips into four, etc.

The FIM strategy (or fimming), is a branch of topping, and got from topping a plant loosely. As opposed to cut the entire tip of a cannabis plant at a fourty-five degree edge, fimming involves pinching off the majority of the cannabis tip with the objective of growing four colas promptly in the spot of one.

Removing Fan Leaves

Removing fan leaves from the plant can be viewed as a training procedure that intends to occupy the plant's vitality into producing bigger colas by limiting the measure of foliage that the plant needs to maintain and increasing the measure of direct light to any development destinations beneath the shade. It additionally diminishes the probability of a vermin or buildup infestation. Notwithstanding, fan leaves do take in light and give vitality to the plant, so cultivators should utilize alert when removing them.

The Cannabis Flowering Phase

The flowering stage is the point at which the female plant produces trichome-secured colas and when the male plant creates and discharges its dust. Cannabis plants blossom naturally during the twelve/twelve photoperiod when the plant gets twelve hours of light and twelve hours of haziness. In nature, sunlight hours are ideal for cannabis plants flowering from July to November in the Northern Hemisphere. On the harvest time equinox in September, the sun is in the sky for twelve hours of the day, with sunlight hours gradually reducing until and through the winter. The inverse is valid in the Southern Hemisphere.

Indoors or in a light-controlled greenhouse, introducing a counterfeit twelve/twelve light cycle will constrain a cannabis plant to bloom.

When Is Cannabis Ready for Harvest?

A female plant is generally prepared to collect when the organs on the highest point of the slim stalked trichomes abandon clear to a smooth white shading. A few cultivators are additionally ready to utilize the shade of the marks of shame to time their collect. Marks of disgrace will in general change from either white to orange or red to dark colored. Producers ought to likewise know about the average flowering occasions of the cultivars they are growing.

Harvesting Your Cannabis

When the cannabis plant is prepared for reap, its valuable and sensitive trichomes are in one of their most powerless states. Overexposure to oxygen, light, as well as warmth may debase cannabinoids and terpenes, or enact them rashly. Trichomes become increasingly delicate and in this manner progressively vulnerable to breaking off the plant whenever misused under outrageous conditions. When harvesting cannabis plants, producers should actualize techniques for drying, trimming, and curing that diminish the measure of fomentation the plant encounters in request to confine any harm to the trichome organs.

Drying

At the point when your cannabis is prepared to reap, cut the entire plant at the base or cut the plant into huge branches. Hang your plant or cuttings topsy turvy on a clothesline in a domain that is not excessively dry or moist. Now, a few producers begin manicuring their plants by cutting off all remaining fan leaves and a portion of the sugar leaves. Plants ought to be left hanging topsy turvy to dry until the stems marginally snap when twisted.

Abstain from losing trichomes by not letting your branches hit any surfaces while hang-drying. Contact with a surface can harm the trichomes and could make them sever the plant. Depending on ecological conditions, the initial drying process usually takes three to seven days.

The trichome organ will encounter a couple of changes during the drying procedure. The most noticable is lost the very sharp smell. This is because of lost the most temperature touchy terpenes, or hydrocarbon aggravates that produce every cultivar's exceptional smell. Studies have discovered that as much as 30% of monoterpenes, or terpenes with two isoprene units (rather than the three isoprene units of sesquiterpenes, four isoprene units of diterpenes, etc) delivered during the flowering stage are lost in the drying procedure. Additionally, when cannabis is dried, terpene mixes are oxidized, and the terpene technically turns into a terpenoid.

Trimming

When the initial drying is finished, it is a great opportunity to finish trimming and manicuring your bud. Cannabis is typically cut to expel the abundance sugar leaves that, while consumable, have a smaller grouping of trichomes than the bloom and can be cruel when smoked. Sugar leaves are not normally disposed of, notwithstanding, as they are amazing for making edibles or concentrates.

Begin trimming by holding your colas by a stem and tenderly cutting ceaselessly any sugar leaves and stems that encompass the buds. This is a sensitive procedure that expects tender loving care. Ideally, this is done over a screen to gather any trichomes that may sever the plant. Take extraordinary consideration when handling your bud. Each snapshot of contact can result in trichome misfortune or harm. At whatever point conceivable, hold your plants and branches before the finish of the stem.

Wet Trim versus Dry Trim

While most cultivators trim their cannabis subsequent to drying, some want to trim while the plant is as yet wet. At the point when cannabis is cut following harvesting, the leaves are still loaded with chlorophyll, which may prompt a determined grass-like fragrance. Trimming the plant once it has lost the vast majority of its dampness is the more conventional methodology.

Curing

Curing can be viewed as the final drying stage, allowing microbes on the outside of the buds to separate any lingering chlorophyll and ensuring the colas are neither too wet nor excessively dry.

This ought to be a continuous procedure, as bud that gets too dry will corrupt all the more effectively during transportation and packaging, lose intensity, and become pointlessly brutal to smoke. Then again, bud that is too wet may develop shape. Preserving aroma and flavor is a key worry for cannabis cultivators while curing. Overexposure to light, oxygen, and high temperatures can separate cannabinoids and terpenes, and at last decrease strength. Striking a sensitive balance among dry and clammy is the key indicator of a finely relieved bud.

Cultivators should never hurry through curing. The procedure regularly requires critical experimentation. One to two months is generally an adequate time span for curing, however inclination and accessible time to fix may contrast among producers. It is critical to keep nature around your cannabis cool during the curing stage.

This curing procedure can be performed by placing your cut buds in a glass container or rubbermaid tote for four two months. During the main week or two, the containers ought to be opened day by day to allow some crisp oxygen to supplant the air in the container. This procedure is called burping and is rehashed until the buds have the ideal dampness content. Over the most recent two weeks of curing the containers are opened each two-three days.

Cannabis Storage Tips

Glass containers are the perfect alternative for transient stockpiling. Ideally, cannabis containers ought to be dark and water/air proof for abundant protection of cannabinoids and terpenes. For long haul stockpiling, cultivators should vacuum seal their final item at whatever point conceivable.

Cannabis development is a committed practice for home producers and expert cultivators the same. To ace growing marijuana takes a ton of tolerance and experimentation, however with time and a couple of incredible proposals from prepared cultivators, you will have the option to give your plants a sound life from seed, or clone, to reap.

Germination from seed is the absolute starting point of life for your cannabis plant. Each suitable seed contains all the information expected to grow a plant simply waiting for the correct conditions to have the option to convey what needs be. Seeds stand by to germinate until three explicit needs are met. Water, right temperature (warmth) and a decent area, usually in a growing medium.

During the beginning times of development, everything the seedling needs is given by the seed itself. Adequate nourishment is provided to last the seed until it has developed enough to begin producing its very own nourishment by photosynthesis.

GERMINATION - THE BEGINNING OF LIFE

Initially, the seed retains water through its husk by imbibition which intends to guzzle or drink. The water hydrates existing proteins and nourishment supplies causing the seed to grow and extend. As digestion gets more grounded hydrated proteins become dynamic increasing vitality generation for the development procedure.

Simultaneously, water increases turgor pressure encouraging cell extension. The principal indication of life will be the cracking of the seed coat and the rise of a small white shoot called a radicle. This rapidly protracts and turns into the tap root. The new tap root pushes down into the develop medium anchoring the plant set up and begins to assimilate water and supplements.

At the same time the new stalk comes to towards the light and leaves begin to shape. The main leaves to show up are oblate, thick and rubbery and are not so much leaves. They are called *cotyledons* and are pre-shaped inside the seed. At the point when hydrated they swell extensively and are utilized to part the seed husk separated and ensure the principal genuine serrated leaves as the crown is constrained up and outwards through the medium.

Before long an extreme change happens called photomorphogenesis. This light-reliant procedure causes the plant to get green and begin photosynthesis.

Various methods of germinating cannabis seeds

Growing cannabis, much the same as different plants, is a natural procedure without an exacting arrangement of rules. It is anything but a linear framework to adapt, however a craftsmanship to be aced. After some time you will build up your very own speculative chemistry dependent on your triumphs and reliably harvest super yields.

There is no single explicit approach to germinate cannabis seeds. Various cultivators will usually decide to utilize one germination strategy that suits them best.

Strategy 1 - IN A MEDIUM

This most intently looks like what occurs in nature. A few producers will plant straightforwardly into an effectively overseen small starter pot or a seedling plate brimming with the medium in which the plant will consume its entire time on earth. This could be soil, perlite, coconut coir or your decision of combination.

As the plant turns into a strapping cannabis seedling needing more shoulder space and root room it will be pruned on into a greater container. Different cultivators will plant the seed straightforwardly into the biggest container straight away in order to keep away from any danger of transplant stun.

The two techniques have their points of interest and burdens. Potting on from a smaller pot risks root harm, transplant stun and all the more extraordinarily root infections. The upside being the plants are simpler to oversee in the beginning times of life when they get considerable consideration with topping and low-stress training.

Germinating in the bigger container risks overwatering and soil immersion in the base of the pot causing molds and green growth. The advantage being up to an additional seven day stretch of undisturbed development.

TO PLANT YOUR SEED:

In the focal point of the pot drive your finger into the saturated medium up to one cm and tenderly spot the seed. Fill over the seed and water into place. It is a smart thought to pack the medium when filling your pots, essentially tap the base of the pot a couple of times on your work surface.

Strategy 2 - PAPER TOWEL

This strategy is favored by the individuals who need ensures about the practicality of their seeds. There is no doubt when seeds have germinated. This gives unlimited oversight over the measure of dynamic space in any develop arrangement.

What you will require:

- Two plates

- Unbleached paper towel

- A plastic sack or cling film

- Clean water

- A warm dull spot

Spot three layers of paper towel on a plate and dampen well by soaking the paper towel at that point draining. Things ought to be wet, yet not swimming.

Spot your seeds onto the dampened paper towel dispersed well. Keep in mind you will require space for your fingers to snatch them when grown and great distancing prevents roots from tangling on the off chance that you confound things.

Spot another three layers of soaked paper towel level over your well-set seeds. Do as such in a manner that gives you a chance to distinguish the edges of the top layer so it tends to be expelled with as meager unsettling influence as conceivable when required.

Presently place in the plastic sack or cover in cling wrap to guarantee stickiness and to prevent the towel from drying out. You can utilize the second plate as a top yet there is a danger of lack of hydration as this is not a water/air proof seal.

Spot in a warm dim spot or on a heating mat. Sprouting time relies upon species. Some quick indicas will be prepared to pot following twenty-four hours. Some different species may take five days. Make an effort not to upset your seeds excessively. Generally, you can see an outline of the root-shoot through the paper towel. Pot your seeds as they grow.

When grown make a 1-1.5 cm profound opening in your chose growing medium, and put the grow root point down, spread over, tenderly water in and place under your vegetation lights. On the off chance that the tap root has twisted around the seed as opposed to being straight still placed it in the medium point down. The seed will do an astute unraveling which helps evacuate the seed husk as it advances toward the light.

There is no compelling reason to go nuts in the event that you have confounded things and the seeds have totally grown. Maybe the tap root has even developed into the paper towel. All is not lost, just now and again. Simply be exceptionally delicate when handling them. Make the gap in your medium as profound as the tap root. They will certainly make due as long as the tap root has not been harmed or broken.

Try to not be crippled if a few seeds do not make it. That is only the manner in which it is here and there and it is not really your shortcoming. On the off chance that it continues happening, audit your procedure or contact your seed provider.

Strategy 3 - JIFFIES AND PLUGS

Different producers select develop fittings or jiffy pots to spare space during the germination time frame. Develop connects have the bit of leeway that they are all set, as of now soaked straight out of the pack and are made considering the cannabis producer. They additionally prove to be useful pre-arranged plate. Be that as it may, they should be utilized quickly or they will dry out.

Jiffy pots or comparative are effectively put away dried out peat pots and should be drenched before using. This has the upside of being ready to redo the supplement and compound condition of the germination medium. Basically add your own witches mix to the water before reconstituting. Plain water is alright obviously.

The two items accompany convenient pre-made openings which are of a profundity without flaw for child ganja plants. They have a level base, stand up simple and are a very basic approach to germinate your cannabis. They have the distinct favorable position of being ready to be pruned on with little root harm and interruption to development. When the main roots are obvious tenderly pot on to an intermediate pot or the final enormous pot. Just drop your seed into the prebored opening and spread it with soil. Spot on a warmth tangle and humidify. Develop attachments and jiffies are additionally similarly as useful for cloning. Simply put your root gelled clone into the pre-prepared opening press and humidify.

PRE-SOAKING IN WATER

A few people like to pre-drench their cannabis seeds before they continue with one of the techniques above. This should be possible by just putting them in a drinking glass of tepid, clean water for twelve-twenty-four hours.

Pre-soaking seeds will mellow the shell and gives the plant an early mini-support. Especially with more seasoned seeds, this is a bit of leeway. More established seeds get a drier and harder skin. By pre-soaking them first in clean water it increases the opportunity to a decent germination rate.

ROCKWOOL STARTER CUBES

Rockwool can be respected and utilized in a similar manner as fittings or jiffy pots. The issue with rockwool 3D squares is more an ethical one than anything to do with their cannabis growing capacity. They are inexpensive, simple to utilize and work well indeed and are utilized widely in the unadulterated hydroponics industry.

Nonetheless, they do not really have the best natural cred as to their production or unimportance. It is hard to think of them as natural that is certainly the pattern in contemporary cannabis request.

Step by step instructions to produce your own cannabis seeds

At the point when we talk about cannabis it is anything but difficult to become involved with the wonderful females that produce those cannabinoid-rich buds we as a whole love and fortune. Truth be told, we have gotten so centered around the female cannabis plants that it is nearly viewed as a terrible sign if a plant happens to turn out male.

Recall that male cannabis plants are similarly as significant as their female partners. Male cannabis plants produce dust like other male plant assortments which germinate female buds to make seeds.

This dust assumes a significant job in breeding as it allows master reproducers to blend and match the hereditary qualities from various plant assortments to make their own cannabis seeds of their own strains.

There are literally a great many diverse marijuana strains accessible. All these strains have their own attributes. It is accordingly imperative to dive into this in advance. Picking the right strain is a significant proces for the home grower. This avoids disappointments sometime in the future.

Do you need the exemplary indica body buzz or the euphoric feelings of an unadulterated sativa? Or do you need a blend of these impacts perhaps? What kind of smell and taste do you like? High in THC or high in CBD? Do you have a great deal of time or do you need a strain that you can collect rapidly?

In our Strain Database you will find in excess of one thousand and five hundred distinctive cannabis strains in sequential order request. Each strain has a portrayal, pictures, and all strain attributes obviously recorded in succession. Because of the surveys you likewise hear an unmistakable image of the point of view of others.

To encourage your inquiry, there is the *Hall of Fame* with all the works of art and other outperforming strains that have given the amazing assortment of hereditary qualities we have available to us today.

In the Top-10 Lists class you will find the ten best strains, each time with an alternate trademark This wide assortment of hereditary qualities is because of the numerous raisers and seed banks around the world.

Picking the right cannabis strain is not in every case simple, especially with such a significant number of strains on offer nowadays. Here you can find a huge assortment of convenient records outlining the Top-10 best cannabis strains in a wide assortment of classes. So whether you are a vet wanting to evaluate something new, a beginner looking for an incredible strain to begin with, or a leisure activity grower looking for a touch of inspiration, you can look at the Top 10 records beneath to find the best cannabis seeds for you.

You can likewise peruse through top item records regarding items other than cannabis seeds. On the off chance that you need assistance finding the seeds that suits you best.

Raisers and Seed Banks

The compelling force of nature gave us the landraces of cannabis sativa and indica that we know under names like Afghani, Hindu Kush, Thai, Colombian and Malawi. Over the years, all raisers around the globe have crossed and tested such a great amount with these and different landraces that a very enormous selection has been made of various strains with a bright combination of smell, taste and impacts.

Right now there are in excess of one hundred raisers and seed banks in our database with a depiction and all their strains. Naturally, the popular organizations are there, for example, Barney's Farm, Royal Queen Seeds, Dutch Passion, Dinafem, Green House Seeds, Subcool's The Dank and Sensi Seeds.

Be that as it may, do not restrain yourself to the enormous brands just, likewise investigate the smaller and lesser-known brands. The majority of them have their own interesting strains which merit significantly more consideration than they actually get. We notice for instance The KushBrothers, Humboldt Seeds and CBD Crew.

Without master cannabis reproducers and seed banks, we would not have the assorted and mixed blend of strains that we as a whole get the chance to appreciate today. Here you can find a rundown of reproducers from over the globe. Find out about what their identity is, the strains they have in their index and obviously their surveys. The universe of cannabis is consistently evolving, and keeping that in mind, this assortment of reproducers is not definitive.

There are literally a large number of various cannabis strains available. While all this assortment implies a lot of decision for purchasers, it can likewise make it increasingly hard to find that one immaculate strain you're looking for. This certainly applies to individuals who are inexperienced with marijuana terminology that can be brilliant with terms, for example, calyx to leaf proportion, SCRoG, Fimming and curing of buds.

Have confidence, on the off chance that you have aced the fundamental principles, at that point you will before long have the option to find your way between all those sativas and indicas.

Here are the best ten uplifting cannabis strains for when you need an uplifting and fiery help

TOP-10 UPLIFTING AND VIGOROUS STRAINS

Cannabis is an incredibly various plant that has been selectively reproduced in a wide range of routes in request to deliver a wide range of impacts for clients to select from. Strains that fit towards the indica end of the range tend to *stone* and loosen up the body, while sativas have an energizing and uplifting impact. The last are extraordinary for recreational fun, and yet they additionally fill in as phenomenal devices for boosting inventiveness and center at work. Sativa-dominant strains have incredible potential for motivating individuals out of feelings of stress and uneasiness.

1. JAMAICAN DREAM

Jamaican Dream is as sativa-dominant a strain can get without being 100% unadulterated. Her uplifting and buzzing high includes won numerous honors inside the cannabis world, including ahead of everyone else at the Slovakia Cannabis Cup in 2011. High THC levels of around 21% and an overwhelming sativa buzz produce a high that is quick acting and incredibly fiery and motivating. This strain is one to move up before working on imaginative tasks, for example, writing, making music, or painting. Taking a hit of this strain before working out or playing sports will likewise help center and sharpness.

The terpene profile within Jamaican Dream highlights mind-blowing kinds of tropical natural product, citrus, and strawberries. These exuberant tastes really work to supplement the energizing idea of the high. Jamaican Dream has a medium growing trouble and is best developed by those with some past experience. She offers stunningly enormous yields when grown both indoors and outdoors, and remains at a medium stature all through the vast majority of the grow cycle. Reap time for outdoor strains happens during October.

2. CHOCOLATE FONDUE

Chocolate Fondue sits immovably on the sativa end of the range, featuring around 80% sativa hereditary qualities. She is the consequence of crossing guardian strains

Exodus UK Cheese and Chocolope, a match resulting in a strain with medium degrees of THC. Chocolate Fondue offers the center ground among smooth and overwhelming highs, making her a fabulous smoking choice on days where you have to remain concentrated, yet need a touch of THC in your life. The high is uplifting and cerebral, with a powerful portion of happiness. Her name gets from the sweet, chocolatey taste that every toke leaves on the taste buds.

The sativa hereditary qualities really appear in Chocolate Fondue's growth design. She grows tall and is definitely more qualified to the outdoors, where plants can grow to their maximum capacity and give immense yields. Whenever grown indoors, expect yields of around 600g/m². Prepare to collect this strain after a flowering time of around eight–nine weeks.

3. OVERLY SILVER SOUR DIESEL HAZE

Overly Silver Sour Diesel Haze is a stunning combination of both the old-school and present day hereditary qualities of Super Silver Haze and Sour Diesel. This strain offers a hard-hitting and ground-breaking high that will fulfill veteran smokers and potentially overwhelm fledglings. The high is incredibly uplifting, motivating, and stimulating. A joint stacked with Super Silver Sour Diesel Haze is an extraordinary wake-and-heat choice alongside some solid espresso to get an occupied and demanding day began the right foot. The blooms of this strain radiate impactful fragrances of citrus and pine.

Very Silver Sour Diesel Haze has a significant distinctive stature to most sativa-dominant assortments, remaining at a medium tallness all through her grow cycle. This smaller size makes her progressively reasonable and a practical alternative for indoor development. Yields are regularly enormous paying little mind to indoor or outdoor development, with a flowering time of as long as twelve weeks.

4. PANAMA HAZE

Panama Haze is oozing with sativa hereditary qualities. With levels ranging from between 90–100%, such a hereditary cosmetics is certain to give the electrical vitality that this cannabis subspecies is known for. This current strain's sativa substance has earned her much prominence within the overall cannabis scene. Such unadulterated hereditary qualities have been passed down from a lineage involving Purple Haze, Green Haze, and F10 Panama Elite. Marvelous breeding has brought about decent THC levels that can reach up to 23%. Such intense degrees of the psychoactive cannabinoid offer an effectively vigorous high that outskirts on hallucinogenic.

Panama Haze puts her hereditary qualities in plain view whether grown indoors or outdoors, reaching towering statures. These weed trees are viewed as simple to grow because of their protection from form, buildup, and brutal temperatures.

5. DESTROYER

Destroyer has not earned its slightly intimidating title in vain. Significant levels of THC work to crush low temperaments and innovative squares. This unadulterated sativa is the offspring of Mexican, Colombian, and Thai hereditary qualities. THC levels of 20% and CBD levels of 1% induce a solid and buzzy high that counters the pressure of everyday life, catalyzing feelings of energy and inspiration. She is the ideal daytime smoke for tedious routines and climbs in nature. The fragrances and tastes of this strain are extremely comforting and refreshing, with lavender being especially dominant within the blend.

Sativa virtue makes this woman grow to colossal statures, becoming the highlight of any polyculture garden. it will contact her maximum capacity when grown outdoors, however can be developed indoors considering space is accessible. She offers medium yields in the two situations and is prepared to collect after a flowering time of as long as fourteen weeks.

6. BRUCE BANNER BX 2.0

Bruce Banner is a reference to the Hulk: enormous, green, and gigantic. These subtleties portray this strain consummately as she really is one of a kind and in any event, intimidating. Bruce Banner BX 2.0 was reproduced in light of just a single thing: unadulterated psychoactive power. Lab results have uncovered that this brute is fit for producing THC levels of up to 30%, creating a high that is stacked with vitality and energy at lower dosages. Higher dosages of this strain are probably going to verge on the hallucinogenic and will certainly be a lot for beginner smokers. This strain is an astounding decision for making edibles in case you're really looking to launch.

Bruce Banner BX 2.0 is a towering sativa that will require some pruning and maintenance. Yields are frequently huge after a flowering time of around ten weeks. Gather time for outdoor plants happens during October.

7. MICKEY KUSH

Mickey Kush is a sativa-dominant woman featuring around 75% sativa hereditary qualities and 25% indica hereditary qualities. She comes from parent strains Jack The Ripper and Sweet Irish Kush, resulting in a strain with significant levels of THC and obscure degrees of CBD. This strain is certainly one that will get you going during the daytime, erasing any feelings of fatigue and procrastination.

Mickey Kush is of medium trouble to develop. She grows to tall statures both indoors and outdoors, churning out medium yields. She has a fairly concise flowering time between seven and two months.

8. JACK THE RIPPER

This dull green excellence ticks all of the crates for an uplifting and stimulating strain. She includes 70% sativa hereditary qualities and has an unpredictable lineage involving Northern Lights, Romulan, Purple Haze, Jamaican Lambsbread, Pluton, and Cinderella ninty-nine. This hereditary mixed drink has created a smooth strain that calms the spirit. Jack The Ripper contains medium degrees of THC, making her optimal for beginner smokers and those needing a light lift for the duration of the day, without becoming overly high. The euphoric and uplifting impacts of this strain are well-coordinated with her delightful tastes of pine, organic product, and lemon.

Jack The Ripper is fairly simple to grow and maintains a medium size all through the grow cycle. This tallness makes her simple to oversee indoors and furthermore includes a component of stealth and protection for the individuals who require it.

9. SANTA CLAUSE MUERTE

Santa Clause Muerte is an unadulterated sativa assortment that produces enormous and thick blossoms that break with psychoactive resin. Her THC level of 20% is sufficient to make even veteran stoners feel invigorated and left. Her parent strains Mexican Sativa and Original Haze have graced her with alluring fruity flavors.

Santa Clause Muerte is viewed as a troublesome strain to grow, and is in this manner best left to progressively experienced cultivators. Plants grown indoors put out yields of up to 600g/m², with outdoor partners pumping out huge reaps and growing to statures of around 2.3 m.

10. FRANCO'S LEMON CHEESE

The flower of this strain are so covered with trichomes that they emit the presence of gems. Franco's Lemon Cheese is a sativa-dominant half and half that highlights 60% sativa hereditary qualities and 40% indica hereditary qualities, making her an uplifting strain that has a component of chill. Her parent strains Super Lemon Haze and Exodus Cheese have gone down aromas and kinds of cheddar and lemon. Her THC levels of 21% are sufficient to trigger a durable and quick acting high.

Franco's Lemon Cheese grows to a medium tallness both indoors and outdoors, offering enormous yields in either setting. She includes a flowering time of as long as eleven weeks and will be prepared to gather during October/November.

Grow lights, sustenance, watering plans, photoperiod strains, bug control, soil quality, hydroponics, drying, curing. From the outset, the universe of cannabis growing can resemble a mind boggling and intimidating spot, and may even be sufficient to put off aspiring growers. Notwithstanding, it does not need to be so difficult or entangled.

At last, cannabis is a weed. On the off chance that you needed, you could give the absolute minimum and still end up with a semi-better than average yield. Proficient growers and veterans in the game invest a lot of cash and time into complex systems to receive the benefits of enormous and top notch yields. In the event that you are simply starting out however, there are numerous things you can do to make matters simpler for yourself when trying to accomplish your first since forever reap.

The cannabis sativa, marihuana or marijuana it is a yearly plant, which means: it germinates, grows, flowers and dies out within a year (aside from in auto-flowering cannabis plants). It is also a dioecious species, that is, there are male and female plants and new samples arise with the cross of the two genders. It is imperative to consider that we will get buds with psychoactive effects just from female plants. The male plants are just used to cross with female plants through pollination.

Most cannabis growers allude to the seedling stage of cannabis plants when the shoots start to build up their first set of *genuine* leaves. Contrasted with the embryonic cotyledons, which have an oval shape, this second set of leaves will as of now look like cannabis leaves with the run of the mill serrated edge, yet it may be one *finger*.

The following leaves the seedling will develop will have three fingers and the following sets that will grow afterward will increasingly more resemble the basic cannabis leaf shape until they will have the full set of five-seven fingers, sometimes more.

TERM OF THE SEEDLING STAGE OF CANNABIS PLANTS

The quantity of leaf fingers, that is the point at which the leaves are finally reaching their final number, is also when cannabis growers say that the seedling stage is finished and the following growing phase of the cannabis plant, the vegetating stage, is beginning. Different growers consider the seedling stage over when the stem arrived at a certain thickness or when the plant has grown three-four leaf nodes.

The term of the seedling stage of your cannabis plant can change depending on whether you develop indoors or out. Developed indoors, your plant will normally spend two-three weeks being a seedling, while the seedling phase when developed outdoors can last as long as six weeks.

While your seedling will develop excitedly to turn into a completely developed cannabis plant, it will spend a decent measure of vitality on developing a root system. A solid root system is significant so that the plant can take in nutrients optimally for sound development.

TIPS FOR YOUR CANNABIS SEEDLINGS

In the event that you place a small fan at the area where you develop your seedlings and have a powerless, however constant stream of air blowing over them, it will profit them in several ways. The airflow can help avoid the development of form, which youthful seedlings specifically are inclined to. The steady stream of air will also make your seedlings put some additional vitality into growing stronger, with a superior and progressively resistant structural integrity.

TYPES OF CANNABIS SEEDS

There are numerous cannabis seeds available. Quickly summarized you can partition these into three groups:

1) Regular cannabis seeds

The plants from normal cannabis seeds can both be male and feminine. In the event that you have requested ten customary cannabis seeds, for instance, you can't know whether the plants will get male or female. At the point when they are developed in great circumstances, you are bound to develop feminine plants.

2) Feminized cannabis seeds

Feminized cannabis seeds are genetically adjusted so that they produce feminine plants in any event 95% of the cases. This forms an incredible favorable position as just feminine cannabis plants produce flowers. The male cannabis plants don't create flowers, contain little THC and can even influence the generation of THC of feminine plants. The feminine cannabis plant produces considerably all the more working substances such as THC, and CBN than a male cannabis plant. Prior to bringing the seeds available, they are first completely tested and further developed so that we are sure that our plants are genetically stable and consistent.

3) Autoflowering cannabis seeds

Autoflowering seeds originate from indica or sativa plants that were crossed with the ruderalis plant. This cannabis plant is situated in areas with short summers. Because of this, the ruderalis plant starts blooming automatically in a short timeframe. (Normally within two or three weeks). The ruderalis cannabis plant is found mainly in Northern Europe, Russia and neighboring countries such as China and Mongolia. This plant contains less THC than the indica and sativa types, which is the reason why they are crossed. The result of crossing the ruderalis plant with an indica or sativa plant is a fast blooming variation with a high THC generation and great flower heads.

4) Medicinal cannabis seeds

Our muscle tensions, ill will course, nausea, spasms, chemotherapy, stress, trouble in sleeping, loss in craving, sexual complaints and hormonal complaints.

Classics new generation - autoflowering

The CLASSICS are the strains of reknown that have substantiated themselves for quite a long time by being at the top for endless decades. A few instances of strains that have a place in this class are White Widow, Amnesia Haze, Super Skunk, Jack Herer, Northern Lights and Cinderella 99.

In any case, these works of art are obviously not works of art if then again not a NEW GENERATION comes up that is anxious to outperform them in enormity. Some genuine instances of strains in this class are: Critical Kush, Zkittlez, Girl Scout Cookies, Jack The Ripper and Gorilla Glue.

Finally, there is the AUTOFLOWERING class. After the introduction of Lowryder Two, autoflowering strains have gotten extremely prevalent because of their particular qualities. A very interesting assortment of autoflowering strains has been made by raisers around the world.

As said previously, there are a large number of various cannabis strains available. This makes it practically difficult to select any 100% address and state-of-the-art list with *The Best Strains*.

Initially, we clearly have not seen, smoked and grown all these strains ourselves. Shockingly we are not unreasonably fortunate. Also, you can obviously ask yourself the inquiry; what is great and what is better? In many cases it just boils down to individual taste and inclination.

So you ought to certainly not interpret these Top-10 Lists as a *we know all*, however consider them to be a decent help for your quest for a specific strain with a certain trademark.

Grow lights, sustenance, watering plans, photoperiod strains, bug control, soil quality, hydroponics, drying, curing. From the outset, the universe of cannabis growing can resemble an intricate and intimidating spot, and may even be sufficient to put off aspiring growers. Notwithstanding, it does not need to be so difficult or confounded.

Eventually, cannabis is a weed. In the event that you needed, you could give the absolute minimum and still end up with a semi-not too bad yield. Proficient growers and veterans in the game invest a lot of cash and time into complex systems to receive the benefits of huge and top notch yields. On the off chance that you are simply starting out however, there are numerous things you can do to make matters simpler for yourself when trying to accomplish your first since forever collect.

Hereditary qualities are the spot to begin. Picking the right seeds to plant will assist you with getting a head start in the basic procedure of growing simple cannabis strains. The main different things you will require are some fair lights, potting soil, nutrients, and water. Goodness no doubt, and some persistence!

1. MANGO SAPPHIRE

Mango Sapphire is perceived as an incredibly simple photoperiod strain to grow. This stunning example is indica-dominant and stems from parent strains OG Kush, Afghani, and Bubba Kush. She offers very strong blossoms stacked with a THC substance of up to 23%. In spite of the fact that her simple cropping nature is fit to beginners, fledglings should at present approach her high with alert. Her belongings are defined by feelings of unwinding, quiet, and sleepiness. She is best smoked during the evening while at the same time watching films and satisfying the munchies with great nourishment. Her high is joined by smells and kinds of sweetness and natural product.

Mango Sapphire can be grown both indoors and outdoors to incredible impact. Indoor plants produce medium yields and remain at medium statures. Outdoor plants additionally produce medium yields, yet detonate to tree-like statures of three m, meaning a decent measure of space is required for this strain. She includes a flowering time of seven two months, with outdoor plants prepared to gather before the finish of September.

2. QLEANER

Qleaner is a sativa-dominant strain resulting from a breeding venture between Purple Urkle, Space Queen, and Jack's Cleaner. This simple strain will remunerate beginner growers with vivacious and enthusiastic sativa buds that produce an euphoric, uplifting, and cerebral high. A THC substance of up to 20% methods this strain is equipped for producing quick acting and durable encounters. Emitting pleasurable smells of sweet organic product, Qleaner is a perfect selection for outdoor exercises, for example, hiking and celebrations, just as parties.

This simple to-grow photoperiod assortment produces medium yields when grown indoors or outdoors. She maintains a sensible tallness all through the whole grow cycle, making her a reasonable choice for those with slightly constrained space. Qleaner highlights a flowering time of between eight–ten weeks, with outdoor plants prepared for gather at some point during October.

3. TROPIMANGO

Tropimango is one of the most delicious simple to-grow strain out there, rewarding fortunate cultivators with intense hits of sweet tropical organic products. This strain inherited her tantalizing flavors from parent strain Somango, which additionally adds to her indica-dominant hereditary cosmetics. Tropimango highlights thick and conservative colas that contain THC levels of around 18%, resulting in an upbeat and quiet high. This strain will help offer some relief from pain and help with achieving a tranquil night's rest.

Tropimango can be grown effectively indoors and outdoors. Indoor plants offer robust yields up to 550g/m², while outdoor plants are fit for churning out a take up to 1800g/plant. Tropimango has a normal flowering time of between eight–nine weeks.

4. SIMPLE SKUNK

It is all in the name with this strain. Simple Skunk has inherited Skunk qualities from unbelievable parent strains Skunk 1, Afghani, and OG Kush. She is likewise a delightfully simple assortment to grow, offering an indica-dominant high when gather time swings around. Simple Skunk has a perplexing terpene profile that outcomes in tastes of cheddar, skunk, and citrus. With THC levels between 15–18%, the high is very mellow and relaxing, offering a soothing body buzz.

Simple Skunk is another photoperiod assortment that is perfect for beginners. She will create medium yields whether grown indoors or outdoors, and her indica dominance guarantees she remains at a reasonable size.

5. GRANDADDY PURPLE S1

This simple to-grow strain is incredibly excellent and extraordinary. She will stand apart from the group in any grow room or nursery because of the incredible purple tints on her leaves and blooms. As an unadulterated indica assortment, Grandaddy Purple S1 offers an incredibly stoning and body-orientated high. Every toke graces the taste buds with kinds of flavor and natural product. Medium levels of THC make her a smooth and relaxed smoke.

Grandaddy Purple S1 highlights a short stature, making her simple to develop in small spaces and ideal for covert development. Both indoor and outdoor yields are great.

6. ALLKUSH

Allkush is an honor winning cannabis strain that plummets from a lineage consisting of Kush and Dutch hereditary qualities. This indica-dominant woman quiets the body and lights the mind, offering loose, garrulous, amiable, and overwhelming impacts. Her aromas are special, described by hints of musk, earth, and sweetness. Her THC levels are high, so don't pack out that bong bowl excessively!

At the point when grown indoors, Allkush plants siphon out a decent 450g/m² and maintain a short stature all through the whole grow cycle. Outdoor plants produce 600g/plant and can stretch to statures of 2.5 m. She makes some flowering memories of around eight–nine weeks.

7. TREATS KUSH

Treats Kush is an intense indica-dominant strain that flaunts a dim emerald-green tasteful. Her blossoms are thick, tall, and column like, with high THC levels that will fulfill even veteran smokers. This honor winning woman is the aftereffect of crossbreeding guardian strains OG Kush and Girl Scout Cookies. The high got from Cookies Kush is incredible, cheerful, and tired, and is increased by fragrances of herbs, mint, and earth.

Indoor yields are around 650g/m², with outdoor yields being huge overall. Both indoor and outdoor plants top out at statures between fifty–one hundred cm, making them tactful and simple to oversee.

8. REGAL CHEESE (FAST FLOWERING)

Regal Cheese (Fast Flowering) is a strain for growers who have a fretful side. She will remunerate cultivators with intense buds within a brief timeframe outline, after around about a month and a half of flowering. This indica-dominant woman comes about because of crossing a photoperiod Cheese with Cheese Autoflowering, allowing for an a lot quicker grow cycle than other Cheese variations. She includes a THC level of 17% and medium CBD levels. Cheddar lovers will quickly perceive her sharp and interesting fragrance, with notes of (shock) foul cheddar and zest. The high is very calming and disposition enhancing.

Regal Cheese (Fast Flowering) can be developed easily in both indoor and outdoor settings. Indoor plants will deliver yields of up to 500g/m² and arrive at statures up to one hundred cm. Outdoor plants produce 600g/plant and detonate to statures of two m.

9. ENORMOUS DETONATION

Enormous detonation is the indica-dominant girl of Northern Lights, El Niño, and Skunk. She includes high THC levels of practically 20%. This culminates in a high that is all the while trippy, relaxing, and opiate. She prods the tongue with contrasting kinds of sweetness, harsh, berries, and flavors. It is sheltered to state that Big Bang brings something new and exciting to the table of simple to-grow assortments.

The strain maintains a short size both indoors and outdoors, yet her yields are the place her name originates from. She will convey harvests that make branches twist. With a flowering time of around nine weeks, outdoor plants will be prepared for the slash before the finish of September. Sow these seeds, and commencement your development venture with a blast.

10. DYNAMITE KUSH

NT Kush is a 100% unadulterated indica strain reproduced to deliver stoning, body-orientated highs with medicinal potential. THC levels up to 22% guarantee instant and dependable highs. She includes amazing tastes of chocolate, cherry, cypress, and almond—a rich, wet combination delighted in by experts and learners the same.

Dynamite Kush is an incredibly rewarding strain for beginners as she is both vivacious and simple to maintain, yet still offers amazing yields. Indoor plants can accomplish around 550g/m², and outdoor plants can create a huge 1kg/plant. This critical range in yield is predominantly founded on how a lot of plants are allowed to extend openly. Indoor plants will arrive at statures of one hundred cm, though their outdoor partners eject to statures of three m.

WHAT IS CANNABIS POLLEN?

Cannabis dust is the same as ordinary dust delivered by different plants.

Dust is fine powder that usually has a brilliant yellow shading. It comprises of tiny infinitesimal grains discharged from the dust sac on male plants.

Dust is utilized to treat female cannabis plants and make seeds. In the wild, cannabis dust is shipped from male plants to females by means of the wind. Be that as it may, in an artificial develop operation cultivators will gather the dust from guys manually and afterward apply it to the females when they have begun developing blooms.

Dust is usually gathered by master raisers and used to make cannabis seeds or breed extraordinary strains. It tends to be manually removed from flowering male plants and put away for well over a year.

HOW TO COLLECT CANNABIS POLLEN FROM MALE PLANTS?

Collecting dust is generally basic. You will realize your male plants are prepared when their dust sacks look full or when you find small fixes of dust on close by leafs.

There are a couple of straightforward approaches to gather the dust from your male plants:

A basic method to reap dust from your male cannabis plants is to delicately evacuate the dust sacs, drying them for seven days, and afterward storing them in a resealable pack (a ziploc sack works extraordinary). When the sacs are dry you can essentially shake the sack delicately and the sacs should begin to part and break, releasing the dust into the pack. You would then be able to evacuate the individual sacs, leaving behind the lovely brilliant dust powder

Another well known approach to collect dust from your plants is to just unsettle the dust sacs so they discharge their dust into a pack or container. You can do this using a ziploc sack; just open the pack, delicately twist the dust sacs so they are practically inside it, and tenderly tap them to discharge their dust. Make sure to evacuate any sacs that may have fallen into the pack or container alongside the dust.

Keep in mind, never go close to female plants in the wake of harvesting dust or having been close to any flowering male plants. Likewise do not keep your male plants in nearness to your female plants or you'll chance pollinating them and destroying your reap.

STORING CANNABIS POLLEN

With regards to storing cannabis dust, dampness is your most noticeably terrible adversary; if your dust gets wet it is literally futile.

The most ideal approach to store cannabis dust is in another resealable pack. You can store dust along these lines in the refrigerator for a couple of days. On the other hand, you can store it in the cooler for as long as one year.

A few people like to store their dust together with plain flour using a one section dust to three section flour proportion. This assimilates any dampness and furthermore make pollination simpler by increasing the volume of the dust gathered. On the other hand, you should have a go at storing your cannabis dust with silica gel packs

At whatever point storing your dust, ensure you minimize the odds of any dampness entering the container or pack. A decent method to do this is to store your dust pack inside one or two different sacks (otherwise called twofold or triple bagging).

USE OF CANNABIS POLLEN

As we referenced before, cannabis dust is typically utilized by raisers and master cultivators to make new strains or seeds. They do this by harvesting dust from their male plants and afterward applying it to female plants that are around twothree3 weeks into their flowering cycle.

At this point, the developing buds on the female plants will have white wispy hairs. These are utilized to naturally gather dust from the wind in nature.

In request to pollinate your plant you will need to apply your collected dust onto the bud locales (usually found where leaves meet the stem of a plant) using a brush. This will make the buds create seeds which can be gathered and developed later on.

Keep in mind, just the bud locales that come into contact with dust will create cannabis seeds. You can decide to apply dust to parts or all of your female plant. You will likewise need to ensure you straightforwardly contact the pistils/hairs on a bud site to guarantee the region is very much pollinated.

On the other hand, you can take a stab at pollinating your female plants using an increasingly *regular other option*. Simply place your male plant in a similar room as a female and give it a couple of good shakes on more than one occasion per day for two-three days. This will help discharge dust into the air and onto the bud locales of the female.

You would then be able to move your pollinated female plant out of the room and again into another develop condition. Simply make a point to keep both your male and pollinated female as far away as conceivable from the females you would prefer not to pollinate.

COLLECTING CANNABIS SEEDS

Cannabis seeds create in the blossoms of the female plants after around four a month and a half from pollination. You will see the seeds starting to shape in and around the pollinated buds.

Pollinated buds appear to be very unique to normal sinsemilla. They usually do not have the same number of rich trichomes and do not shape into huge colas. Instead, they are usually smaller and much progressively bulbous.

a month subsequent to pollinating your female you can begin checking in on your seeds to check whether they're prepared for reap. Essentially choose seed from a pollinated bud; develop seeds will have an incredibly hard shell and be a dim darker or tan shading. They may likewise have some light striping on the external shell.

On the off chance that your cannabis seeds do not meet this depiction, let your plant build up somewhat more.

Some cannabis plants can create develop seeds really late into their flowering cycle. On the off chance that that is the situation, ensure you keep your plant buzzing with a lot of light and supplements.

When you are convinced your seeds are full grown, essentially collect your buds and uncover in profound to get all those excellent seeds. You can store cannabis seeds in a cool, dry spot for at any rate a couple of years or germinate them to begin growing new plants right away.

THE FUNDAMENTALS OF GROWING CANNABIS

Growing your very own weed is the initial step to becoming a genuine cannabis epicurean. Fortunately, cannabis is a significant simple plant to develop. Be that as it may, on the off chance that you need some great outcomes it is important to do some exploration first.

Starting a develop will assist you with building a solid association with the cannabis plant, and really comprehend what this excellent plant is all about. You have to realize what cannabis plants need in request for them to develop into solid develop plants that convey great measures of lovely and rank buds. To give these necessities, most cultivators need to do a few arrangements first.

Cannabis is a plant, and simply like any plant, it requires four basic components to flourish:

- Light

- Water

- Nutrients

- Fresh Air

On the off chance that you can suit every one of these components, the chances of growing solid, sound cannabis plants with a pleasant reward toward the end are incredibly high. How about we experience every one of these components:

LIGHT

Light is fundamental for photosynthesis, the essential work attempted by plants. Sunlight (or fake light) gives the fuel to plants to develop, assimilate nutrients, and in particular, create damp buds. The light spectrum and term of introduction should be balanced for both the vegetative and flowering stages. Cannabis cultivators frequently state *all the more light = more bud*.

The Importance of light for growing cannabis

Without the sun, there would be no life on earth. Plants blossom with sunlight and need it to fuel their development and direct their life cycle. What is more, cannabis is the same.

Light is the way to photosynthesis, a procedure which cannabis (and most plants) use to develop and create solid root frameworks and foliage. Also, enormous, fat buds.

Photosynthesis involves three key parts: light vitality, consumed by the plant's leaves; water, ingested by means of the plant's roots; and carbon dioxide, assimilated from the air. Plants utilize the vitality they assimilate to essentially use water and carbon dioxide, which they at that point use to develop.

Without light, plants cannot photosynthesize and will eventually pass on. Thus, it is essential your plants get a lot of light for the duration of the day so they can develop and eventually produce flowers.

Other than photosynthesis, light is likewise key in keeping plants in their vegetative development stage and additionally forcing them to flower when they (or you, the cultivator) are prepared. Cannabis is a photoperiodic plant, and thusly, will flower once it gets twelve hours of uninterrupted light and twelve hours of complete murkiness. Now, plants automatically *think* they are approaching the finish of summer, which is the point at which they naturally flower.

THE LIGHT SPECTRUM

To all the more likely see how cannabis plants utilize light, it comprehends the light spectrum.

There are essentially 7 kinds of light that make up the noticeable spectrum; violet, indigo, blue, green, yellow, orange, and red. These sorts of light usually sit within a wavelength of 380nm to about 750nm. Light somewhere in the range of 280 and 315nm is known as UVC and, aside from causing burn from the sun, is likewise reputed to increase THC levels in cannabis plants.

Paces of photosynthesis are most noteworthy in red light, trailed by blue light, and at last green light. Ideally, you'll need to utilize various types of light during the vegetative and flowering stages of the cannabis life cycle:

• **Vegetative stage:**

For vegetative development, it's ideal to utilize blue light (which usually lounges around 400–500nm). Blue light will enable your plants to grow a lot of sound leaves and thick, solid stems. Using more grounded lights this right off the bat in the game will bring about your plants stretching out and becoming hard to oversee.

• Flowering stage:

During the flowering stage, it's usually prescribed to utilize red light (usually between 620–780nm). These lights will enable your plants to grow enormous buds and best emulates the common point of sunlight during pre-fall/early harvest time.

Various types OF GROW LIGHTS

In case you are planning an indoor develop, you have seen that there is a gigantic assortment of growing gear accessible to you. The following is a waitlist of the absolute most normal sorts of develop lights utilized by cannabis cultivators.

• Fluorescent lights:

Fluorescent lights have a lower wattage than most other develop lights. They are generally intended to be utilized to develop plants that require lower light intensities than cannabis. There are two main kinds of bright lights you can use to develop; smaller glaring lights or CFLs (small, *wound* looking lights), and T5s (long cylindrical lights, usually accessible in a board).

Glaring lights are incredible for cultivators on a limited budget or those working in tight spaces, as they are anything but difficult to install and usually don't occupy as a lot of space as different sorts of lights. Shockingly, bright lights won't really carry out the responsibility once your plants flower, despite the fact that they can be helpful for the seedling and veg stages.

• HID lights:

High-intensity release (HID) lights are another well known alternative for cannabis producers. They are controlled by huge bulbs which usually arrive in a wide range of shapes and examples. While they produce a lot of incredible light and can deliver amazing outcomes, they are known to get exceptionally hot.

Henceforth, most producers using HID lights will likewise utilize exhaust frameworks to remove a portion of the warmth from their develop space. Some regular sorts of HID lights include high-pressure sodium (HPS) and earthenware metal halides (or CMH).

• LED lights:

LED develop lights are significantly more dominant than fluorescent or HID lights. Be that as it may, they are additionally (usually) considerably more costly. Driven lights are known to run a lot cooler than HIDs, and most expert LED develop lights will accompany some kind of inherent cooling framework.

They are frequently simple to set up and put your plants at a far lower danger of being scorched. LEDs are additionally penetrative, meaning they don't should be moved as regularly as HID or bright lights, which will spare you some physical work.

THE RIGHT AMOUNT OF LIGHT FOR YOUR GROW SPACE

At the point when cannabis plants finish their seedling stage and enter the vegetative stage, they need in any event two hundred and fifty watts/m² of light to develop appropriately. For greater, quicker development, you'll ideally need to surpass this sum and give around four-hundred-six-hundred watts for every m². On the off chance that you need to take it to the maximum, you can consider growing with one thousand watts develop lights for every square meter.

When growing marijuana indoors with these kinds of lights you need to keep an eye out for too high temperatures. These lights make a great deal of warmth, especially the six-hundred W and one-thousand W lights can transform your develop room into a sauna.

Lighting System Design Principles

A decent lighting framework will bring about both more significant returns and lower vitality utilization. In any case, what is beneficial for one business may not be useful for another, and plenty of choices can make selecting the correct lighting framework for your cannabis activity confusing.

For instance, the correct lighting configuration relies upon variables, for example, the ideal light intensity level, the design of a development domain, the accessible stature and the light conveyance of the luminaires. In addition, practically all agriculture lighting organizations will give light plans. However not all know or pursue great structure principles.

Along these lines, on the off chance that you intend to depend on the suggestions of a lighting organization, or on the off chance that you need to begin without any preparation yourself, it is important to acclimate yourself with some fundamental lighting principles. Here are eight principles to kick you off.

1. Determine your objective level of light intensity.

The ideal objective level will rely upon the growing technique, plant stage, cultivar and power costs. Our examination, just as research led by the industry, recommends that level might be more than double the light gave by a twofold finished, one-thounsed W HPS installation. In this way, in case you are growing in a greenhouse in the U.S. or then again Canada, chances are that the sun isn't providing enough light to develop cannabis optimally the vast majority of the year. You ought to determine what the lighting shortage is in January, the darkest month. You will have to install enough lights to make up for that shortage, except if you are eager to forfeit yields during times of the year with lower characteristic light levels.

2. Position lights to maintain even intensity over the shelter.

Spotlights at statures and in areas comparative with each other so you give, by and large, your objective light intensity to the shade while minimizing variety in that light intensity. To explain, imagine every one of your lights is a showerhead that splashes water (i.e., light) onto your plants. At the point when splashes (i.e., light emissions) from various showerheads cross one another, more water hits those spots. You will likely place those showerheads with the end goal that each plant gets near your objective level. Obviously, a few plants will get hit by more water, yet you can put the showerheads with the end goal that those distinctions are minimized.

3. Purchase a quantum sensor.

You can just assess a lighting framework's plan and enhance it on the off chance that you can gauge the measure of light the framework conveys to your overhang. Quantum sensors allow you to gauge the number of photons that fall on a specific area each second and that are within the wavelength go that plants use for photosynthesis. The unit of estimation of light intensity is called photosynthetic photon motion thickness (PPFD). Lux, lumens and foot-candles are misleading measurements when dealing with plants since they are measures dependent on what a human eye sees, which is not a similar spectrum go that plants use for photosynthesis.

4. The state of your growing space matters.

For instance, plant lighting research from Cornell University has indicated that if your growing space is formed like a square shape, staggering your lights is bound to improve the appropriation of light, and yet that is not the situation for square-molded develop spaces, which, examine has appeared, are bound to profit by lining lights up in lines.

5. Try not to belittle the expense of blocks.

Think cautiously about the position of fans, crossbeams, ventilation socks, and other potential lighting obstacles. Their shadows, which are practically unperceivable to the eye, can decrease the light intensity by about 10% in explicit areas. A general dependable guideline is that a 1% decline in intensity compares to a 1% decline in yields.

6. Light-intensity variety

is regularly lower toward the focal point of a room and increases as you advance toward the border.

One approach to increase consistency at the edges of your develop space is to diminish the separation between lights (or increase their intensity) around the border. Actually, light conveyance and vitality effectiveness can be improved by placing lower-wattage lights toward the focal point of the room and higher-wattage lights toward the edge.

7. Comprehend that the plants will do some work for you.

Inevitably, when designing a room or imagining enhancements, sooner or later, extra upgrades to light dispersion will turn out to be extravagant. In any case, plants will consistently do a portion of the work for you. For instance, plants will change the morphology and edge of individual leaves to utilize accessible light more proficiently, however, it is hard to see that plants are doing that. So when you are considering increasingly complex changes to your room configuration in request to improve light appropriation (e.g., making lights versatile), inquire as to whether that investment will include enough improvement above what the plants will do themselves to make the investment justified, despite all the trouble.

8. Comprehend the Inverse Square Law.

You can increase light-intensity consistency by increasing the separation between the plants and the lights, but since of the Inverse Square Law, small changes in separation will bigly affect normal light intensity. Think about the showerhead model. As you increase the separation between the showerhead and a container on the floor, you decline the measure of water that falls inside the basin and increases what arrives outside of it. The photons created by your light carry on along these lines, to a degree that relies upon the state of the light's focal point. As you increase the separation between the lights and the plants, you increase the measure of light that spreads out and hits things like walkways and walls. In this way, there is the capacity to increase PPFD and vitality savings by moving lights nearer to plants. One of the essential advantages of light-emitting diode (LED) apparatuses is that you can draw them nearer to plants on the grounds that an LED's light shaft spreads less and it creates far less brilliant warmth. Simultaneously, as you draw the lights nearer to the plants, you increase the changeability of light intensity over the room. Imagine moving all the showerheads two inches from the floor. A few spots would get a great deal of water while others would get none. Finding the ideal point in that exchange off is maybe the most focal component of an ideal lighting structure.

WATER

Water is the lifeblood of almost every living being on planet earth. To keep your plants in shape you have to know how, when and how much water to give them. The sum and recurrence to give water rely upon the hereditary qualities you use, your develop technique, atmosphere, and obviously the size of your plant.

How and when to offer water to your cannabis plants

The lifeblood of almost all living beings on earth, water is crucial for your cannabis plant's endurance. In view of that, knowing when and how to water your cannabis plants is fundamental for keeping them in ideal shape.

Despite the fact that cannabis will show flexibility with an absence of, and in many cases, an excess of water, neither one of the states ought to be delayed. In doing along these lines, cultivators risk poor bud creation and hindered development. In more terrible case situations, the absence of both water and nutrients could cause your cannabis plants to bite the dust.

For by far most of the cultivators, watering in the morning is the favored alternative. When daylight or fake light starts, cannabis plants will utilize the water and the nutrients gave to direct photosynthesis, in this manner driving development.

In the event that there is not any water accessible when this procedure begins, cannabis will be adversely affected, similarly, we would be entirely futile on the off chance that somebody requested that we start work with no nourishment or drink already.

When in doubt of thumb, water promptly in the morning on the off chance that you are growing outdoors. In the event that you have decided to develop indoors, give your cannabis plant water when the lights-on cycle begins. Thusly you will guarantee they have enough access to experience the most intensive piece of the day.

GIVING WATER TO YOUR PLANTS

Do you douse the whole plant, liberally soak the topsoil, or spray a light mist? It may not seem like a major distinction, however, the system you choose will direct how much water to give. The best technique is nothing unless there are other options. Ideally, for most regular structure root advancement, water cannabis plants through base feeding.

By placing pots into a plate of water, the roots will draw what they need upwards through the topsoil. It also encourages your roots to develop downwards, which is useful for the entire plant.

In the event that after thirty mins there is still water remaining, expel the excess. In the event that there is no water left, add somewhat more to see on the off chance that it is absorbed. Because of the novel process of osmosis, root structures will just ever take the water they do not require anything, more, nothing less.

In the event that base feeding is impossible, saturate your substrate by adding water to the top until you see it draining out the base. Try not to water so a lot of that a pool remains on top or the soil becomes sloppy. You need to soak the whole substrate, however you're not trying to suffocate it.

The water should generally drain away when you have moved onto the following plant/pot. Getting the measure of water right can be troublesome until you have a vibe for how thirsty your plants are. Just stick to adding a smidgen at once until the water drains and you feel it is satisfactorily hydrated.

Drip feeding water by means of a water system is another strategy that is profoundly proficient. Albeit all the more challenging to set up, it takes a great deal of the complications and risks out of watering by hand. We will cover the benefits of this technique later.

HOW OFTEN SHOULD YOU WATER?

Watering recurrence is a slightly increasingly complex variable. The rate at which you water will fluctuate according to temperature, the strain's attributes, regardless of whether it has started to flower, and even the size of the leaves.

The easiest, all-around approach is to water each two–three days, depending on the soil and the intensity of your lighting hardware. Soil can dry out, and as a general rule, it almost should. On the off chance that your soil or some other substrate you are using is forever wet, this can urge shape to develop and cause roots to kick the bucket.

Push a finger knuckle profound into your substrate to measure how hydrated it is. In the event that the substrate feels dry and your cannabis is not a dynamic shade of green, at that point watering is likely required. In the event that, then again, the substrate is still moist, hold off! Your cannabis will survive, and it is far easier to add water than it is to remove it.

Weight is another telling variable of whether your plants need watering. In the event that you are growing in pots, get every container you intend to water. In the event that it feels heavier than usual, again, hold off. There is still water present, so no further moisture is required. As a point of reference, fill an unfilled pot with a substrate so you can think about the general load of dry versus wet.

ADDING NUTRIENTS

Adding nutrients to water is straightforward. Ensure you pursue the maker's guidelines and blend altogether. In the event that you know the nuances of the strain you are growing, it is now you will modify any supplement concentrations. At the point when you are content with the solution, apply to the soil as you would a customary watering.

Numerous episodic accounts like to see between 10–20% water spillover into the trays underneath the plants. The hypothesis is that this will help keep supplement lockout from occurring. Just like with plain water, an excessive number of nutrients can be inconvenient.

Diverse water sources

Straight from the tap is the place most growers get their water. Assuming those same growers approach the rest of the variables of growing cannabis with absolute precision, it seems a shame that some do not think about the complications tap water creates.

Depending on your area, the mineral substance of tap water differs uncontrollably. This, with regards to mixing nutrients, can make calculations precarious. A simple method to balance the uncertain idea of tap water is to fill a basin and leave it to rest medium-term.

The following day, you should have the option to take a progressively exact reading, and in most cases, the water should be suitable for use. In the event that you realize you live in a territory with incredibly hard water or elevated levels of sulfur, there are several testing kits alongside synthetic remedies to bring the water to an increasingly stable composition.

Another advantage of leaving water to rest medium-term is it will be at room temperature. Water that is excessively hot or too cold also does harm to your cannabis plants.

Checking the ph value of water

Prior to testing the pH of your water, pursue the step listed above and leave the water to rest medium-term in request to diminish the possible chlorine content.

When you have done as such, you will require the following: your water, pH here and there, a pH meter, and your nutrients. On the off chance that you are going to use a watering can, at that point have that prepared as well. The solution blended in the can should then be transferred to the watering can.

With all gear close by, your objective pH for water should be 6.3-6.7 for soil and around 5.5 in the event that you are using a hydroponics setup.

Include your nutrients and either the pH up or down until you get the right reading. Just make a point to stir altogether for the most precise recording.

CONTROL THE TEMPERATURE OF YOUR MIX

As simple and sham as it might sound it is very significant for plants to get a solution within an ideal temperature zone.

Cheerfully most of the growers do not run into problems of this nature, however consider this story as a lesson. One of our companion growers spent around five weeks last winter trying to make sense of what was the issue with his plants.

He checked different elective solutions, gear, lightsource, changed the feeding schedules dramatically at some points to analyze and so on; just until he understood that the tap water coming out of the wall had a lot of lower temperature in the winter (15-17C) contrasted with the summer season (+25C).

He viably soaked the plants with too chilly solution making them stress increasingly more not being ready to absorb necessary nutrients. In the event that your water/supplement blend is beneath 22C, plants probably won't have the option to absorb Phosphorus and different elements appropriately.

USING A DRIP IRRIGATION SYSTEM

We alluded to this before, however *drip watering through a water system is a definitive solution to little and regularly*, waterings, allowing growers more noteworthy precision over how much water their plants get. You should append the water system to a supply of water, setting up drip points at the base of each plant.

The whole system will be encouraged by the main supply pipe, which shouldn't be any more distant than fifty m. from the water source. Drippers connected to painstakingly set t-junctions along the main supply pipe will be responsible for providing the plants with water.

Pursue the same principles as previous methods of watering, allowing the water to quickly gather on the surface of your substrate at that point drain away. Because the distribution of water is slow and controlled, it is unmistakably progressively hard to fall into the snare of overwatering.

As drip feeding water is much slower, you should change watering times so that you start the process prior.

When working with drip water system systems, make sure to keep them clean and stay away from knockoffs. Most problems occuring while at the same time working with drip system originate from absence of legitimate maintenance and modest hardware. Make sure to clean the tubens and connectors all the time to keep away from them getting stuck and risking ruining your crops.

THE DANGERS OF OVERWATERING YOUR CANNABIS

In spite of the fact that it is usually amateur growers who commit this error, overwatering is a troublesome propensity to defeat for some cultivators. Our desire to give the best to our cannabis plants can make us overzealous with the resources it needs.

As well as water, roots need oxygen. In the event that your root system remains doused continuously, oxygen is inaccessible, and your plants cannot develop. The cells in the roots will kick the bucket thus also will the remaining plant structure.

Additionally, excess water can prompt root decay, shape, and mold, all of which will, again, kill your plant or harbor bacteria that will do likewise, just after some time.

Luckily, overwatering is an easy mistake to spot, most of the time plant looks like its wilting while the pot is soaked with water; shockingly, the main cure other than waiting for it to dry out is to transfer the plant starting with one pot then onto the next containing fresh, dry substrate.

On the off chance that root spoil has settled in, ensure you remove all influenced areas before replanting. Barely any companies offer solutions for root problems. In some cases, advantageous funghi or symbiotic bacteria can abstain from running into these problems.

WHAT HAPPENS WHEN YOU DON'T GIVE CANNABIS ENOUGH WATER?

Leaves will start to shrivel and turn inwards, root structure will shrink, and plant structure will begin to bow through absence of strength. Left long enough, your plants will bite the dust with no water, just like humans, animals, and all different plants would. Without the nutrients gave by the water, all of the plant's normal processes like photosynthesis will slow or stop.

Drawn out periods of dryness will eventually cause perpetual harm to your plant, resulting in stunted development and poor bud generation. Nonetheless, short periods of dry spell are easily helped by giving plants water in the *little yet frequently* way. At the point when you are sure they are re-hydrated, normal watering cycles can resume.

NUTRIENTS

Notwithstanding light and water, cannabis plants need an assortment of nutrients. On the off chance that you go to a develop shop and search for 'All-In-One' supplement bottles you will most likely quickly see the following three-letter combination: N-P-K. This represents the proportion of nitrogen (N), phosphorus (P), and potassium (K), the three elements of sustenance cannabis plants use in enormous quantities. Nutrients can be either natural or synthetic.

The Full Guide to the Best Cannabis Nutrients

Cannabis plants actually use the process of photosynthesis to change over light into vitality. The marijuana cultivator must know about this key factor, as obliviousness of this reality leads numerous to the fake conclusion, that massive doses of synthetic fertilizers are the best way to secure an overwhelming weed harvest.

Numerous variables must be considered in request to select the correct cannabis nutrients and administer them at the perfect time. Your decision of cannabis strain to crop and development strategy are the two most significant elements.

The objective is to integrate the fitting fertilizers for the development medium and apply in doses suitable for the specific cannabis strains.

CANNABIS BASE NUTRIENTS

The three letters you will see prominently displayed on each brand of cannabis nutrients and supplements are the N, P, and K values. This represents the proportion of nitrogen, phosphorus, and potassium respectively.

Base nutrients are the essential compost feeds, that the producer will add to water to advance it with the macronutrients and, gave it is a quality item, most of the necessary follow elements like calcium, magnesium and a host of other required micronutrients.

In simple terms more N is desirable during vegetative development, with low levels of P and K. As cannabis plants transition into the flowering stage, P and K must steadily be increased, while N is gradually drained, swinging the ratios the opposite way. That is the reason base nutrients come in separate blends for specific use during vegetative development and sprout.

Soil growers can usually stick with plain water for the first two-three weeks, as even light blend soils have sufficient quantities of both full scale and micronutrients to nurse an infant cannabis plant in any event through the seedling stage and into vegetative development.

Be that as it may, hydroponic and coco cultivators should include base nutrients at roughly 25% strength from at an early stage in the develop, as the medium is not pre-treated and inert.

To maintain a strategic distance from overfertilisation of cannabis seedlings, numerous such growers will start their beans off in pre-treated rooting cubes, that just require plain water until roots begin to distend from the 3D shape, indicating it's the ideal opportunity for a transplant.

CANNABIS SUPPLEMENTS

Cannabis supplement supplements are of incentive to incorporate in each producer feeding schedule. Unless you are an outdoor natural purist, that mixes their own super soil to grandmaster producer standard, at that point you have to pay attention to supplements.

Supplements can assume a job in the whole cannabis life cycle. Gainful parasites and microorganisms like mycorrhizae can be inexpensively added to rooting medium to advance the improvement of a solid root zone.

From the earliest starting point, when the cannabis seed germinates, it will be urged to root well, as the mycorrhizae will shape a symbiotic relationship with the root zone.

Enzymes are perhaps the most significant supplement to include all through vegetative development and the sprout phase. These catalysts successfully serve to open the maximum capacity of your cannabis plants.

Besides, enzymes help the root zone to flourish and encourage the absorption of the full scale and micronutrients. Frequently neglected and excluded from feeding schedules, yet enzymes really are fundamental.

Fluid silica is one more pivotal cannabis supplement, especially for hydro growers. Adding a light week by week dose of silica all through your plant's lifecycle is an incredible precaution measure to avert a host of nasty pests and pathogens.

Silica strengthens the cell walls and is the best method to toughen up a cannabis plant. Vigorous solid plants are less susceptible to disease and the feared bud decay is less liable to strike cannabis plants siphoned up on fluid silica.

Natural molasses can be found economically in most supermarkets and it is actually a cannabis super-supplement wealthy in follow elements. Nothing keeps the microorganisms in soil more joyful. Not so much a possibility for hydro growers, as it's sure to stop up something.

Yet, for the natural cultivator, we suggest you make molasses your new best companion. Fantastically successful in the later blossom stages to assist resin generation and virtually guarantees full season buds.

Sprout boosters

Cannabis sprout boosters are the place the producer must discern. Some strains respond to a specific brand of sprout booster and not all that well to an opponent organization's item. Different strains don't really require these products at all.

As you become progressively acquainted with various cannabis strains and gain all the more growing experience through experimentation, you will choose which item best suits your develop operation. A lot of anything can be a terrible thing and an excessive amount of P and K will consume buds as opposed to boost creation.

FOLIAR FEEDING

Marijuana can also drink up nutrients through its leaves and foliar feeding is a genuine alternative until the plant starts to develop buds. The best time to apply a foliar feeding is within the first two hours of the light cycle to anticipate the wet leaves getting light consume blotches.

Truth be told, it is best to spray down the underside of leaves as much as possible and do not become really excited soaking the plants or shape could be an issue.

For outdoor growers fresh air is a simple thing to fix. Notwithstanding, when growing indoors, it is crucial to manage real air stream. Plants use carbon dioxide from the air to make nourishment and sugars. The oxygen from the air is used for breath (breaking down nourishment to make imperativeness).

Give your cannabis plants enough fresh air

There are numerous variables that influence how cannabis plants develop. The most predominant worries for growers usually involve light, stickiness, and nutrients.

Notwithstanding, one often ignored factor that can hugy influence your final assemble is air course.

In this book, we are going to look at the significance of giving your cannabis plants fresh air. Besides, we will likewise look at some central ways you can make airflow in your develop space.

HOW PLANTS USE OXYGEN

Much the same as individuals, plants need oxygen in request to persevere.

During the day, plants will take in carbon dioxide from the air, water from their roots, and imperativeness from the sun to convey sugar, a wellspring of essentialness both of them can use and store. This technique is called photosynthesis.

At whatever point a plant does not move toward enough sunlight it will eat up the sugar it has made in request to remain alive. In any case, in request to separate that sugar into a usable essentialness source, it additionally needs to consume oxygen.

While plants naturally produce oxygen when they mix, they additionally take in extra oxygen from the earth to help advance development in regions that ca not photosynthesize, (for instance, the roots of the plant). This method is called breath.

THE IMPORTANCE OF FRESH AIR

In request for your plants to develop to their most outrageous potential, it is indispensable they have consistent access to fresh, oxygen-rich air.

Fresh air generally contains between three-hundred-five-hundred sections for every million of carbon dioxide. The perfect conditions for cannabis plants is around one-thounsend-one-thounsed and fourty-hundred sections for every million.

Presently, in outdoor develop situations, this is not usually an issue, as air is always circulating. Nevertheless, in an indoor situation, things can get somewhat precarious, especially in case you're growing various plants in a confined space.

To ensure there is sufficient fresh, oxygen-rich air in your develop district, we prescribe investing in a normal ventilation structure that moves old air out of the earth and brings in fresh air from the outdoors.

Ventilation systems can be as straightforward as two or three strategically set fans or as cutting edge as an exhaust structure. What heading you go relies upon your inclinations, budget, and how judicious you need (or need) to keep your develop movement. We'll look at a part of these various systems in more detail later on in this post.

THE IMPORTANCE OF AIR CIRCULATION

Air dissemination is a surefire way to deal with ensure your cannabis plants approach a great deal of oxygen. Notwithstanding, that is not using any and all means the main inspiration driving why it is significant.

As a matter of first significance, genuine dissemination is basic for minimizing the peril of bud spoil and various conditions.

Exactly when plants inhale, they produce water which usually develops along the leaves and buds of cannabis plants. An advancement of this dampness is one of the main sources of bud rot and various conditions, for instance, shape and form.

Genuine air dissemination allows air to blow over and around your plants and evacuates dampness, consequently reducing the threat of the above conditions.

Air dissemination likewise encourages you shield your plants from garden bugs like bug bugs and development gnats. These nuisances experience trouble living in all around streamed zones and generally search out territories with torpid air.

In addition, the airflow will likewise dry out the top layer of your plants' soil, which makes it harder for bothers like gnats to breed.

By having air hover all through your develop district, you're likewise help to keep mugginess and temperatures enduring all through the entire condition. This is basic for greater develop operations, as stale conditions can make hot and soggy pockets, which can influence the development of individual plants.

Finally, exposing your plants to circulating air likewise encourages them create solid stems, which proves to be useful when they start flowering and need to help the heaviness of the buds.

HOW TO GIVE YOUR CANNABIS PLANTS FRESH AIR

FANS

Fans are a generally reasonable and straightforward way to deal with keep air moving around your develop zone.

Ideally, you will have to keep air blowing both above and under the main shade of your plants. From this time forward, we suggest one fan over your plants and one underneath the main shade.

We additionally prescribe using oscillating fans as they are modest to run and can make a good, even breeze all through a decently wide domain without blowing an excess of air on one single plant.

At the point when you've installed your fans, ensure you check your develop zone to see that the breeze is unfaltering all through. Additionally, pay special mind to indications of wind-consumed leaves that are rolled and twisted under in request to look "tore at."

EXHAUST SYSTEMS

Exhaust systems are considerably more modern than a straightforward fan framework, but at the same time are significantly more costly to install and maintain. Notwithstanding, they allow you to expel old, dormant air from your grow zone and causes your plants grow to their maximum capacity.

Exhausts are usually installed over the overhang of your plants as sight-seeing rises to the highest point of the room. Many grow lights additionally accompany exhaust expansions, allowing you to install the exhaust pipe directly close by your light.

The thought here is straightforward; while the fans in your room help to flow fresh air, the exhaust hauls out any old air.

Be that as it may, installing these systems is significantly progressively unpredictable and requires a strong understanding of the airflow in your grow zone. You will additionally need to figure the vital quality for your exhaust fan, especially in case you are running a huge grow operation, and substantially more.

What Is A Mother Plant?

A mother plant is a plant so great that fresh cuttings are taken from it to become precise hereditary copies. Taking cuttings instead of growing seeds leads to an increasingly consistent crop in terms of intensity and finishing time. In any case, these mother plant *clones* can still display variations in phenotype. An interesting plant with uncommon qualities is usually chosen to turn into a mother plant.

With suitable consideration, you can continue to keep this plant alive for anyplace between six months and three years, and past. This could be a cost-successful solution for your development operation. Mother plants are a perfect method to source cuttings of your preferred weed. Discover the craft of growing and maintaining flawless mother plants with Royal Queen Seeds.

At the point when you find a strain that rocks your reality or eases your pain, you will need to encounter it again and again. The easiest method to rehash a most loved discovery is by taking clones from mother plants. Using mothers has various benefits. Characteristics are known and repeatable, females are ensured, and development and supplement profiles are standardized. Mothers can be kept alive indefinitely when well-maintained, and delighted in for quite a long time.

THE BENEFITS OF USING MOTHER PLANTS

At the point when coordinated right, cloning from mother plants can mean harvesting one day and having more plants all set the following. With overlapping growing schedules, you can always have plants in flower, with increasingly prepared immediately.

Mother plants are perfect sources for infant plants when using the sea of green (SOG) procedure. Similar-sized clones will make a homogeneous overhang with no tall or short phenotypes to consider.

Mother plants can be as large as you need them to be. Ambitious grows with lots of space will require enormous mothers for lots of clones. Smaller spaces that can just fit a couple of plants will just require a small mother plant. Cannabis can be easily controlled to suit your personal circumstances.

Consistent characteristics are ensured without fail. Business growers value the standardization; domestic growers welcome the dependable presentation.

There is no risk of males with clones, making for a productive develop space filled exclusively with females.

WHY AND HOW TO RAISE YOUR OWN CANNABIS *MOTHER PLANT*

Cannabis plants originate from one of two sources: a seed or a clone. When talking about cannabis breeding, *mother stock* typically refers to a profoundly esteemed plant that growers take clippings from to make clones, which are genetically indistinguishable cuts that can be re-planted to develop another plant.

Mother plants develop in a continual vegetative stage as clones are over and again cut from her. Taking clones guarantees that all the plants in your nursery will develop at generally the same rate, produce a similar quality item, and develop with the same power as the mother they originated from.

WHY ARE CANNABIS MOTHER PLANTS IMPORTANT?

Cannabis mother plants ensure consistency, and this is key for growers who are required to give an item that customers request on numerous occasions.

When growing from seeds, growers need to manage undeniably greater inconstancy in development patterns, supplement needs, and different attributes. While some stable seeds produce less of this wild diversity, you may still make some hard memories achieving the even shelter you'll find with clones.

Cannabis mothers will also save you time and cash. Premium seeds cost upwards of ten dollars a pop, and purchasing individual clones can also get pricy. Instead of buying seeds each time you need to grow another crop, germinate a bunch of the same seeds and select a mother based on the criteria discussed beneath. A quality mother plant will give you quality clones over various seasons.

SELECTING A MOTHER PLANT

Mother plants begin their life as clones. You should set aside a region separate from the flowering room. This mother plant home will be kept in perpetual vegetation mode. On the off chance that you as of now have a separate vegetation space, you are set. If not, you should make one.

Making mother plants requires some readiness when the original plants are developed from seed. It is a cautious game. Each plant in the develop should be cloned. These clones should be plainly related to their source plant. After the source plants have been flowered, harvested, dried, relieved, and consumed—that is the point at which you settle on a decision of which one to keep.

Keeping itemized records and pics of development characteristics and effects ensures things don't get confused. Choose the most outstanding plant from a single-strain crop or the best of a multi-strain crop. By week two of flowering, males will have uncovered themselves and can be disposed of.

MAINTAINING MOTHER PLANTS

Three things are essential information for good mother plant upkeep:

- Appropriate topping

- Air pruning roots by hand or with air-pots/develop bags

- Permanent vegetation cycle

When customized for the size of your develop operation, solid mother plants will give an endless supply of virile clones of your preferred strains.

Treat your mother plant as you would treat some other vegetating plant. As it is developing, just use weakened nutrients and increase the strength as the plant grows. Flush them consistently with unadulterated, clean water or flushing solution to avoid supplement lockout. Ordinary maintenance will ensure a long, sound life for your mum.

TIP-TOP TOPPING TIPS

Clone size is space-subordinate. Fifiteen cm cuttings will strike well overall, as will five cm and anyplace in the middle. A mother plant that provides long cuttings will take up substantially more volume than one that provides smaller cuttings. Enormous operation, huge mother; small operation, small mother.

There are two types of mother plant. The perpetual plant and the transient plant. Perpetual plants are topped, tied, and controlled to give a continuous supply of clones. Transient mothers are cloned from the present plants under vegetation, before being placed into flowering. As it were, each plant replaces itself before it goes onto the blossom phase. This way, there is no requirement for a separate plant. Try not to stress, there's nothing of the sort as hereditary float. Your lone stress here is that clones may fall flat and plants could be lost.

There are as numerous sound mother plant topping techniques as there are ways to develop cannabis. In the domestic situation, the home-growing hobbyist is generally going to have eight weeks between the requirement for plants to blossom. Considering a two– multi week time span for cloning and vegetation, this is five weeks or a greater amount of mother plant arrangement.

You can top once, tie the parallel branches level as they develop, at that point clone from the fresh doublet of branches that develop from every hub—leaving two branches to rehash the process. Continually topping the apically dominant branches will result in a bushy plant with many clone sites to choose from. Bonsai-ing also makes for a decent selection of branches while keeping the mother size leveled out.

AIR PRUNING THE ROOTS

Air pruning the root system is necessary vandalism for continued mother plant wellbeing. At the point when customary solid-walled pots with drainage holes in the base are used, plants eventually become pot-bound. Roots will bunch and spiral around the pot and eventually succumb to decay or strangulation.

Air pruning involves cutting the root ball down to 33% of the original volume, at that point repotting. Fresh roots will at that point develop and plant improvement continues, liberated by sick wellbeing. It is best to air prune a couple of days after clones are made. Plants have recouped well and the lesser foliage will have less interest for nutrients from the convalescing root system.

Air-pots and develop bags close up apically dominant root shoots with a thin film of air as they search their way through the develop medium. This prevents the roots from reaching the edge of the pot, and thus allows for more weeks in a single pot—as opposed to root-trimming once every month or somewhere in the vicinity, as with normal pots.

Eventually, the pot will top off with an excessive number of huge, fat roots and structure a hitched root ball. This leads to an inefficient surface region, which in turn inhibits appropriate supplement take-up. Now, numerous growers will begin another mother plant.

In the two cases, in the event that you are unsure of the root state of a plant, sit tight for a couple of hours in the wake of watering when the excess has drained away well. This will ensure the develop medium does not collapse in your grasp because of being excessively dry or saturated.

Upswing the pot and tenderly expel it to expose the subterranean workings of the roots. In the event that roots can be seen starting to pursue the shape of the pot, the time has come to air prune. In the event that roots are not visible, just as tenderly supplant the plant. Focus on disturb the roots as little as possible.

Indications your plants may be pot bound?

•   There are signs of supplement consume and deficiencies simultaneously.

•   Plant development slows considerably and they lose their power.

•   There are general signs of sickness or pH imbalances that don't respond to amending.

In the event that your mother plants are responding strangely following quite a while of solid development, overturn them and inspect the root system.

ALWAYS VEGETATING

Mother plants should be kept in the vegetative phase of development. This means they should get over twelve hours of light for each twenty-four hours. On the off chance that they are in a vegetation chamber, they will get the standard eighteen/multi day/night vegetation cycle. On the off chance that they are in their very own space and you are wanting to slow development rates, a fourteen/multi day/night cycle will keep them in vegetation, yet growing slower. On the off chance that you need more clones as speedy as possible, keep up the eighteen/six for quick development.

The same rules apply for keeping a mother plant vegetating as for general vegetation. A metal halide light to exploit the blue spectrum of light promotes perfect vegetation. Use legitimate veg nutrients. On the off chance that you are growing organically, the medium will be supplanted each air prune to ensure consistently accessible nourishment.

Mother plants are an extraordinary method to accomplish consistent quality and execution from your preferred types of cannabis. At the point when given the correct consideration, they can create clones for quite a long time.

HOW TO SELECT A CANNABIS MOTHER PLANT FROM SEEDS

Because clones are genetically indistinguishable from their mothers, selecting a quality mother plant is significant to a successful harvest. While a pack of seeds may all be the same strain, there are always various phenotypes (distinctive physical expressions).

Some plants express several distinct phenotypes, which can make selecting a mother progressively troublesome. Others may deliver somewhat more consistency, which simplifies the selection process. Regardless,

The best way to selecting a quality mother is as follows:

- **Step 1:** Germinate the seeds.

- **Step 2:** Wait until the plants show their sex in vegetative development, and afterward take a couple of clones from every female plant. Make certain to name which seed they originated from.

- **Step 3:** Let the clones continue to their flowering stage while keeping the original plants in vegetative development.

- **Step 4:** As the new plants flower and are harvested, observe traits like smell, season, yield, bud structure, and development design.
- **Step 5:** Take the corresponding original plant from whichever clones you loved most. This one is your new mother plant.

The Most Effective Method To Protect Mother Plants

An initial step that some farmers take to secure their mother plants is germinating and growing them in a natural base.

By starting out natural, you allow your mother plants to develop resistance to battle diseases as opposed to protecting them with strong non-natural mediums and nutrients, said Cody Erickson, head cultivator of the Khush Kush in Bellingham, Washington.

You will also need to use the original plant from seed as your mother plant as opposed to the first clone she created. Plants developed from seed are known to have stronger, more profound tap roots than those of their clones notwithstanding stronger resistant systems.

Not far off, you can use nutrients specifically created for mother plants that advance strong clones while keeping your mothers solid as clones are over and again cut from her. You will need clones taken from plants with strong cell walls and high starch levels. Nitrogen-rich nutrients result in fast development that leaves the plant with thinner cell walls and a lower density of carbohydrates. Instead, use nutrients that have a higher level of calcium to help bind cell walls and increase the density of carbohydrates. These carbohydrates and water stored in the clone will be used by the plant to deliver roots.

Instructions to Preserve Cannabis Mothers

Mother plants have a life cycle, just like all living beings. Indeed, even with meticulous consideration, your preferred mother plant will show diminishing returns after some time. The clones taken will develop with less power, produce lower-grade cannabis, and leave you reminiscing of more promising times.

This can take a year or two to happen, and keeping in mind that that seems like quite a while, it is best to store seeds from the plants you're at present growing so that when the opportunity arrives, you'll be prepared to start over with the same genetics you love.

HOW TO CLONE WEED

Cannabis can be imitated asexually or sexually. Asexual spread is what is known as *taking cuttings* or *cloning*. Numerous growers exploit this awesome process known as cloning. Simply stated, the cloning process is when development shoots or branches are expelled from chosen giver plants and induced to frame roots in a separate develop medium. By taking cuttings from a mother, each and every clone will be an ensured female plant. A nursery can be sustained indefinitely by taking cuttings before plants begin to flower.

To enable you to out, here are the cannabis seed banks that work in any nation.

Cloning offers growers numerous benefits. For one it allows them to have a constant supply of female plants, by using clones, a producer has a sound, steady supply of ensured female-just plants. A clone is a precise hereditary copy of its parent. So, you can use your most vigorous and intense plants to use as mothers, and each clone you take from it will be vigorous and powerful as well. Clones will always keep the same sex and energy of the mother plant. It is also possible to make a nursery of plants that will last for quite a long time through cloning from a single female *bonsai* mother plant.

INTRODUCTION TO CLONING

Mothers (or *Bonsai Mothers*) can be kept alive for quite a while to continue to deliver sound offspring, at the same time, the more you keep it alive the more it has the opportunity to fall prey to insects, form, parasites and disease.

Cloning is a famous simplified strategy for replicating your plants. To clone marijuana is to take a *cutting* from a growing branch tip and root it. Cloning is by a long shot the most effective and beneficial means of cannabis engendering for

growers, both indoors and outdoors. The best time to make and use clones is the point at which you have an extraordinary interesting plant whose specific hereditary code merits preserving and perpetuating. Consistency is a typical development objective

among quality cannabis growers. Since indoor cultivator's usually cannot dedicate existence to plants that may have very various habits in development, flowering time, or yield, clones offer the upside of uniform genetics.

Uniform genetics simply means that your plants will be the same tallness, have the same development habits, will mature and flower at the same specific time, and have the same power, taste, fragrance, smell, traits, and so on. They will also respond to the same outside stimuli in the same definite fashion (such as fertilizer, lighting, bending, cutting, stress, and so on). Sooner or later the cultivator will at that point know precisely what to do to his crop to ensure a quality, substantial harvest unfailingly.

The benefits of creating a nursery of genetically indistinguishable cuttings from a specifically supported mother plant will allow you to deliver a consistent, known quality and amount from each plant and expect that all plants will develop at the same time. This guarantees the same consistent, quality, harvest from consecutive crops (as long as the same top notch clones are used for planting) This strategy is CRUCIAL for business situated weed farmers.

Hereditary consistency works the two ways however. This means if your chosen stock plant is lacking strength, wellbeing, harvest weight and so forth; it is clones will come up short on those traits as well. That is the reason choosing solid parent plants is essential.

On the off chance that you find a seed strain you really like with an awesome hereditary profile, you can keep it indefinitely by cloning her effectively. You can make literally 100's of solid female plants from one single mother. Cloning is extraordinary for those growers who have little cash to spend on numerous seeds.

Cloning has the additional advantage of reducing the time it takes for a plant to develop. Clones can flower as soon they arrive at twelve inches, so cloning can shorten the absolute growing time (which normally takes ninety – one-hundred-thirty days from seed to harvest) to just ten days. In this manner, cloning allows the cultivator to plant THC intense plants that will continue to develop into full strength at a quick rate.

A one month old rooted clone acts precisely like a multi month old plant and can be activated easily to flower by using the twelve/twelve photoperiod.

A remarkable plant can be revived and cloned considerably after it has flowered and been harvested! In the event that a small measure of vegetative issue is left growing on the base of the plant and it is set under an eighteen hour light cycle at that point all the little nuggets will stretch into vegetative shoots, which may then be cloned and developed into a full mother plant, which would then be able to be cloned indefinitely. This will give you many uniform harvests of your preferred plant.

When using clones for regenerating, your nursery can be designed and used most proficiently because you know the plant's definite growing habits. Also when business growing, since the plant's qualities are known, you can establish an interminable income age cycle appropriately. The downside to clones is that they can be tedious to get ready and are subject to overwhelming disappointment rates.

WARNING: It is basic that you take clones from a mother plant as it were. Taking clones from clones may cause the plants to suffer from *hereditary float* and structure mutations or undesirable development characteristics.

Growers regularly will make clones from their plants when they are still in their vegetative development stage (cuttings are made easier while the plant is still in its vegetative development stage). This technique for propagating development asexually to ensure consistency in development, yield, and consistency is very well known nowadays.

STARTING FROM SEEDS VS CLONES

Numerous amateur growers ask: *"should I start from seed or should I develop clones?"*

Growers regularly face the decision to begin their development from seeds or rooted clones. There are distinct advantages and disadvantages to both. The customary method to begin growing another marijuana plant is to plant seeds. About portion of the seeds will form into plants that end up being male. The males are then expelled from your nursery and the remaining females will be of varying quality. Be that as it may, shouldn't something be said about clones? Allows just say you get an amazing female plant that you presently need to continue to deliver. How would you do it so that you can develop out future generations of precisely the same indistinguishable awesome plant consistently, producing a constant progression of incredible buds? This is known as recropping and is the strategy for obtaining a second indistinguishable harvest from the same plant. The answer, of course, is to take a cutting (clone) of the desirable female mother plant. This is the best way to get a uniform crop.

Growing from clones means that you will harvest more bud sooner. Numerous individuals who start a nursery nowadays know someone who will give them a couple of clones for the simple pleasure of sharing something to be thankful for. Some individuals sell clones just, regularly growing an exclusively vegetative nursery while never flowering.

These clone aficionados keep an assortment of select mothers from excellent strains and develop them on a continuous eighteen hour light cycle. They can take in substantial income selling trays of cuttings, either rooted or simply fresh cut. Rooted clones are more expensive than fresh cuttings.

In the event that you approach someone who grows, you can ask them for some clones, as this will be the easiest method to obtain them. On the off chance that you don't approach any clones, you will, at that point need to purchase seeds as referenced previously. Some individuals sell specific strain clones just, utilizing an exclusively vegetative nursery while never flowering their bud. They can make great cash selling trays of cuttings, either rooted or freshly cut. Rooted clones are undeniably more desirable than fresh cuttings.

I suggest growing from seeds so you can choose the specific plant that suits your needs, thus you can select the best *pioneer* plants. Ensure when you are starting from seeds to take two clones from the base of each plant directly before putting the plants into the flowering phase of development. Keep them alive, and watch future generations soar.

It does not make any difference which develops system you use, you will undoubtedly use clones sooner or later. They can significantly improve the proficiency of your growing zone, and are a fantastic method to preserve your preferred plants.

Advantages of Starting With Clones:

•   An astounding approach to keep a steady supply of plants around.

•   Saves a huge amount of time.

•   Guarantee of having a female plant.

134

- Clones are a lot faster to veg up and flower than starting from seed, resulting in a speedy harvest and an a lot shorter turnaround time.

- Clones can be immediately developed into mothers and re-cloned, for an instant vegetative and flowering crop

- Since indoor growers usually can't dedicate reality to plants that may have very various habits in development, flowering time, or yield; clones offer the upside of uniform genetics.

- Clones are genetically indistinguishable, however some differences will still be apparent in the phenotype. As a rule clones will show even development and uniform growing characteristics.

- Rooted clones can be flowered quickly if space or time is an issue.

- Clones can rapidly furnish the cultivator with a strain's characteristics (smell, life, branching example, Sativa/Indica dominance, rooting quality, and so forth).

Disadvantages of Starting With Clones:

- Genetic consistency means similar resistance and susceptibilities to insect assault, disease, microbial infections, supplement deficiencies, and some other kind of weakness the parent plant may have that normally would be less.

- Likely to hurt the plant had it been reproduced of various varieties. As it were, degeneration is probably going to spread all the more rapidly.

•   Lack of assortment. Clones from the same parent will all taste very similar and make precisely the same high. This is ideal for business growers seeking uniform standardization development to increase profits on a huge scale, however, most smokers growing their very own cannabis will in general favor various varieties of the pot.

•   Clones can be hard to find. Clones from obscure sources are of suspect quality and questionable hereditary predisposition.

•   Growers run a high risk of inheriting problems from the last cultivator: Root decay, spider mites, fine buildup, and so on. On the off chance that these problems are not distinguished and treated, they can immediately spread to a whole crop (and nursery)

•   Unhealthy clones may pass on or remain in shock for an all-encompassing period.

•   Availability. Shipped clones might be in shock and take weeks to recuperate. There are countless loathsomeness stories of restorative clones shipped with no security and showed up a level.

•   Clones are more light-sensitive and fragile than seeds. Clones set aside an effort to get established, and are easily singed by excessive light (and nutrients). They require more consideration and care in the early development stages.

•   As clones are almost always female, breeding options are constrained. Bisexual advancement is always possible with unstable clone crosses.

Advantages of Starting With Seeds:

•	Seeds obtained from respectable seed banks are of known lineage and genetics. You will have a reasonable thought of what the strain will do in terms of yield, quality and flowering time.

•	Your seeds should create sound plants, free of disease and pests.

•	Hybrid power. Females developed from seed are frequently higher yielding than clones. Strains can lose their energy after some time; growers might need to revive they are developed with the same successful strain.

•	Breeding and crossing options are possible with male seeds. (Feminized seeds produce a higher level of female seeds, yet 100% female is never ensured.)

•	Gives growers more power over advancement and selection.

Disadvantages of Starting With Seeds:

•	Problems with ripoffs, shipping/customs seizing seed bank deliveries, switched seeds.

•	Cost. Seeds can be expensive, per seed pack, however, in the time they take to create a flowering crop.

•	Unstable crossover strains.

•	Not all seeds will be reasonable (germinate) and just half of the unfeminized seeds will be female (feminized seeds may create up to 90% females).

•	It may take many seed packs to discover an incredible mother.

•   Seeds take quite a while (and there is more work, cash and time involved) before a harvest can happen.

•   The final results are uncertain.

•   Indoor producer's usually cannot dedicate existence to plants that may have very various habits in development, flowering time, or yield.

CLONING IN PERLITE AND VERMICULITE

Perlite and vermiculite, combined at a 1:1 proportion, make a compelling, modest, and generally accessible cloning medium. Simply blend half perlite with half vermiculite, include enough water so it's moist, and fill your small containers. Ensure you keep your medium moist. Wash/rinse any new perlite with ~pH 6.0 water to evacuate any dust residue before use when cloning.

Step 1. Set up your mother plants in any event 6 hours ahead of time with a fresh drink of water so they are completely stacked before you cut.

Step 2. Using a screwdriver, toothpick, or outsider probing gadget, make a small gap in the medium, around three cm profound at each clone site.

Step 3. Take the growing tips from the mother you wish to spread with sharp scissors – they should associate with six to nine cm in length.

Step 4. Remove all leaves aside from the main one or two, plus the small growing shoot.

Step 5. Recut the stem end with a sharp X-acto or scalpel, making it as calculated as possible for huge surface territory contact and water take-up.

Step 6. Optionally dunk the cut end into a rooting hormone containing fungicide.

Step 7. Cautiously insert into the growing medium, tenderly patting the opening closed.

Step 8. Spot containers in spread plate and spread with dampness arch. Spot prop plate on heating cushion set to *low*.

Step 9. Hold under fluorescent lighting, misting them every day for the first scarcely any days if your atmosphere requires. You may need to lightly water the medium on more than one occasion before roots show in seven to fourteen days.

There are diverse *grades* or sizes of perlite and vermiculite. For cloning, the small to medium perlite and the medium to huge vermiculite are best, yet do not stress on the off chance that you cannot find the precise size you are looking for. The fifty/fifty blend holds water rather well when there are no plant roots sucking it up, so do not overwater your cuts.

The Simplest Cloning Method Known to Man

As easy as cloning is to the masses that use powder, fluid/gel rooting hormone, bubblers and soil, and so on, there is an even less mind boggling strategy for cloning that is so easy, it must have been around for a considerable length of time, if not centuries. The main ingredients involved are water, light, and the cutting you might want to root. In the following model, you can see cuttings of three distinct sizes of clone.

The first with two leaves and a single growing tip (S). The following has four nodes, yet at the same time just a couple enormous leaves (M). The third is 6" tall, has seven nodes and several sets of good-sized leaves (L).

As with typical cloning, you promptly dunk the cutting in the water for around fifteen to thirty seconds, tweaking it to dislodge any air bubbles that might be present.

However, the biggest contrast is, you won't expel the cutting from the water until it has roots huge enough to support the foliage above. Ensure the cup, which contains the cutting, is obscure. This prevents the light from shining legitimately on the roots.

The cool thing about this strategy is the lighting system. Cloning using this technique works 100% of the time simply by sitting cuttings on a windowsill that receives no immediate sunlight. Truth be told, slightly shaded would be stunningly better. In the evenings (short days), you can sit them on an end table more than seven feet from a ceiling mounted one-hundred W incandescent bulb. At sleep time, just mood killer the lights like typical, and when you get up in the A.M. Spot them back on the windowsill. During the more drawn out daylight hours they can be left on the sill full time. Be that as it may, recall, no immediate sunlight.

M and L have scarcely an inch of water to sit in. Any more and it would cover one of the leaf stems. The smaller one stayed in the plastic because the stem was too short to even think about sitting in water and stay upstanding in the cup. Do what's necessary to keep at any rate ½ of the stem in the water.

Notice the glass that diffuses light, an additional measure against an excessive amount of light exposure.

The clones developed roots at far various speeds. S showed in seven days, with a small ¼ long root and another small protrusion.

When (S's) roots arrived at this degree of improvement (nine days), (L) was just putting out the first nubs that would be roots. (M) has shown no inclination of rooting at all. It boils down too the thickness of the stem. Both (M) and (L) have the same size stem however (L) has unmistakably more foliage on top.

Transplanting Clones

In around three-five weeks your cuttings will frame a solid root structure. Around then the time has come to transplant them to a bigger container so that their root structure can extend out and become much further. Ensure there is a lot of air in the development medium, as this will significantly upgrade solid root development.

Following this, in around one-three weeks, root structure should be grown enough so that the cuttings can be put straightforwardly under a HID. You will at that point take your female clones and spot them in a bigger growing medium. Transplant just the strongest, vigorously-rooted clones. The lights will be found just a couple of inches over their tops. Keep them growing in vegetative (following the light cycle as suggested in the guide) and afterward flower them when prepared.

For best results and to ensure a substantial, frosty harvest; do not transplant clones until they build up a dense solid root system. Signs that clones have rooted include yellow leaf tips, roots growing out of drain holes, and the vertical development of your cuttings.

Note: When transplanting be extremely cautious with the fragile roots.

Transplanting is significant as soon as plants exceed their containers. This is because plants with cramped root systems will become sickly, stunted plants.

Attempt to keep the develop mediums the same to anticipate plant transplantation shock. On the off chance that you are using rockwool to transplant into soil, you have to direct moisture levels for ideal results. Let your rockwool 3D shape dry out just enough whilst keeping the soil moist so that the roots will enter into the new growing medium in search of moisture and nutrients.

Note: For best results, water your clone with a half-strength bacterium vitamin B complex (such as trichoderma) around two days before you transplant.

Transplanting Clones 1

Step 1. The first step is to set up your new container. Fill a 2.5/3 gallon container with quality potting soil. Top it off leaving about ~2 inches between the soil and the top edge of the container.

Note: When cultivating a Bonsai Mother she will require a bigger container, somewhere in the range of 10-30 gallons is perfect in the event that you intend to keep her for a year or more.

Step 2. Treat your new develop medium by watering it with a quarter strength quality hydroponic fertilizer solution until your develop medium is sufficiently rich and saturated. Ensure the solution drains openly out of the base.

Step 3. Set up a gap (use your best judgment depending on the original growing medium and root ball size) in your container.

Step 4. Carefully pop the root ball out of it is container. An easy method to do this is flip around the container placing your hand over the top with your fingers in the middle of the stem, flip the container over and slide it off allowing the root ball to sit in the palm of your hand. Be very mindful so as not to disturb the sensitive roots!

Step 5. Delicately set the root ball into the readied opening inside the new and prepared container.

Step 6. Pack around and fill soil around the root ball.

Step 7. Water. For best results, blend a half-strength fertilizer that ideally contains trichoderma bacteria or vitamins(B). You need your soil to be extremely wet, yet draining uninhibitedly.

Step 8. Spot your plants close to a light source. At first a HID is excessively intense, to cure this simply place your container at the fringe of your nursery or under a screen. Following a few days of decreased intensity light your plants should begin to look strong and solid, they will at that point be fit to be moved under full light.

ROOTING HORMONE

Rooting hormones extraordinarily speed up cell level plant processes. When a stem is taken and needs to create roots in request to continue the plant's survival, it has to adjust and transform from producing green stem cells to manufacturing new root cells. Rooting hormones enliven this process tremendously. As soon as you make your first cut, clones begin to naturally make these hormones and send them to the injury. This takes about seven days.

At the point when you dunk your cuttings into a rooting hormone it will fill in the need until characteristic hormones dominate and significantly speed up development. While dipping, give them a five-ten second plunge. Napthalenaecetic Acid (NAA), Indolebutyric Acid (IBA), and Dichlorophenoxyacetic Acid (DPA) are three substances that stimulate this process and incredibly assist in root cell creation. Search for a business rooting hormone that contains all three (on the off chance that you can find it) of the above ingredients.

Note: When mixing and you have to find out the ppm (parts per million) of your rooting hormone, simply duplicate the rate listed on the item by 10,000. For instance, if your item says it contains .8% DPA, it contains 8000 ppm DPA.

Another extraordinary ingredient accessible in numerous products today to assist in clone rooting is known as trichoderma bacteria. This bacteria when introduced to your clones will cause the roots to become faster and the bacterium also assists them in absorbing nutrients better.

In the case of using a spray, gel, or other type of rooting hormone make a point to adhere to the instructions cautiously. When spraying make certain to use just enough, don't spray your clones so a lot of that their leaves are dripping with rooting hormone.

Willow Tree Water

In case you are looking for a stunt to create incredible speedy vigorous root development when cloning, you have to obtain regular Willow (tree) Water. There is a substance inside of all willow trees that promotes incredible root development. Imagine those tremendous enormous trees with their massive profound root systems.

At the point when willow water is used on your tiny little clone's root systems and blended in with business development hormone, it produces unfathomably awesome results. You will be shocked at how fast and how vigorous your clones roots create.

To make your willow tree water compound is easy! Go to your nearest Willow Tree and find branches that were developed this year. They should be around 1.5 inches in breadth. Evacuate any leaves and cut the stems into 1" lengths. Spot as huge numbers of these little cleaved willow stems as you can inside a glass or a quart container. Soak them medium-term for twenty-four hours in distilled water. In the wake of soaking, spill out the willow water to use it for an incredible rooting hormone.

For best results, simply soak your clones in the willow water rooting compound for twenty-four hours, at that point plant into your rooting medium. When using a business rooting hormone compound, substitute the willow water instead of normal water in the blend.

Variety: Willow Rooting Hormone Tea

Cut some willow branches (all willow species produce this characteristic rooting hormone), into 2" or 4" long pieces. You should slice enough pieces to fill a bowl.

Put the willow cuttings into a major pot (or pot) on the stove, load up with water (all cuttings should be secured by water). Turn on minimum warmth setting, spread with a cover, and leave on low (yet don't bubble) for two hours. At that point turn off warmth and leave pot secured for twelve hours.

After the blend has cooled for twelve hours, the willow water should be a dim dark colored. Strain out the willow water, and discard the branches. Empty the blend into a container with a plastic top with holes pre-made, and just drop your cuttings in. Give the clones a chance to sit in the hormone for twelve to twenty-four hours (thus allowing the cuttings to completely absorb the rooting hormones), at that point plant into your medium.

Use as a lot of rooting hormone as you require, at that point discard the used segment. The unused hormone can be stored in the cooler for quite a long time.

Cloning Devices

At the point when you take cuttings and are prepared to transplant you are going to require some sort of gadget to keep your delicate clones in ideal conditions until they develop strong roots. Obviously will you put them straightforwardly into a medium? And yet then what?

Here are a couple of devices used for this purpose:

Two Liter Bottle

This is likely the cheapest and easiest consistent technique to root a small number of clones. Just cut the base 40% off a two liter soda bottle, put a clone in rockwool or an entire small container with another medium inside the base. Spread with a plastic pack and hold the sack down with an elastic band. Before sealing give it a puff of breathed out air to fill it with CO_2. This traps stickiness inside, it is typical and desirable for moisture to condense on the container. You should trade air each day until roots show up.

146

Moistness Dome

The most widely recognized device used is the moistness arch. These can be purchased for ~ten dollars-fifteen dollars at any hydroponic develop shop.

They consist of a plastic plate that is just the correct size for a sheet of small rockwool cubes to fit inside of. There is then a reasonable plastic spread that fits over the plate to trap stickiness. Depending on the number and size of clones you should trade air between one-three times every day.

Miniaturized scale Bubbler

These can be purchased or constructed.

Essentially a bubbler consists of a plate with a spread. In the spread, there will be numerous net pots and inside the plate will be water and aquarium air stone strips. The strips bubble air through the water causing the bursting bubbles to moisten and oxygenate the medium in the net pots. These can be used with or without a stickiness arch spread. On the off chance that a spread is used air trade is required according to a simple.

Wick Cloner

These simple and productive cloners are generally constructed as opposed to purchased. A system similar to the bubbler is used with a plate and spread. Instead of net pots the plate has half pint plastic containers suspended over the water. A wick, usually a 1½ " bit of shoelace or strip of fabric, at that point goes from an opening in the base of the container down into the water. The containers are then loaded up with perlite. The wicks maneuver up moisture into the perlite. An arch spread is not used with this technique.

After you take your cutting and safely pack it into its new growing medium home, the work isn't finished. This is the most sensitive piece of a clone's life, this is the basic stage that determines the wellbeing and force overall of your small developing plant.

To what extent Clones Take To Root

After about seven days you can test to see if your plants have started to root. Evacuate the stickiness vault and leave it off for between twenty minutes and two hours. Watch the clones for any signs of wilting while the vault is expelled. In the event that the plants have not withered at all, at that point they presumably have enough root advancement to support themselves. In the event that no shrink is seen leave the arch off, on the off chance that they are shriveled, spray the cuttings and vault and supplant the arch on the plate.

When you have determined that the plants can support themselves, stop misting the cuttings and leave the moistness vault off.

WARNING: Once the plants have roots, constant misting can actually be unsafe to the plants (and can cause shape.)

Are you most likely wondering what measure of light is necessary to ensure the clones greatest and fastest rooting time right? Well I will let you know. Clones root the quickest with eighteen-twenty-four hours of Fluorescent light. As previously mentioned, it has been frequently suggested by cutting edge growers that you should not use a HID light immediately, however on the off chance that you must (on the off chance that you do not approach fluorescent lighting), place the plants on the edge of your nursery so they get less intense light. You can also shade them with some sort of fabric or screen, this works equally well.

Your cuttings are sensitive at first. To ensure they wont shrivel, keep them in a zone that gets just a moderate measure of light. Give the clones a chance to stay in a six/eighteen (six hours of light on, eighteen hours of darkness), in a smaller scale hothouse for the first two days of soft fluorescent light. The darkness stimulates the clone to develop roots instead of spending precious vitality and resources on photosynthesis.

Spot the fluorescent cylinder six inches over your clones for ideal light exposure and development upgrade. Direct light will consume them because without roots the stem can't supply the leaves with enough water to coordinate the leaves' pace of transpiration.

Note: When using fluorescents, a combination of both cool white and warm white are most amazing for rooting.

Try not to move clones underneath intense brilliant light until they have completely built up their root systems!

Fertilizers

When rooting, clones require minimum amounts of nitrogen, and significant levels of phosphorus. This will enormously assist in promoting fast vigorous root development. Precisely following five days your cuttings should be prepared with a high phosphorus fertilizer. Weaken it to ¼ of typical strength, once every week.

The way to getting a 100% consistent clone survival rate is to rehearse your cloning method until you get it absolutely flawless, down to the precise measure of fertilizer at precisely the same time, including the same handling strategy and light exposure/moisture levels and so on. It takes practice, yet with time and following the tips outlined in this guide, youwill get it sooner or later.

A typical cultivator mistake is to think more is better. This is NOT the case with fertilizing. Over-feeding your clones will significantly hinder and slow down root development. Following the recommendations above is bounty.

Note: you might need to use a root complex during the growing phase of your cuttings. A root stimulator is an ideal starter for the cuttings. It activates the plants to grow thick stems and a solid root system.

Temperature

Cold cuttings may never root. On the off chance that the temperature at clone root level is less than 65°F (18.3°C), you'll need to use a heating mat. Temperatures of around 75-80°F (23.8-26.6°C) will advance the best development.

The ideal pH level to support the best possible vigorous root development in clones is between five and six.

Watering

Watering clones is easy! Just plunge them in a lightly prepared (around 100-200ppm) water, or cause your own watering to can! You can use a standard plastic waterbottle with holes jabbed into the top.

Plant roots development is significantly upgraded by oxygen. Circulate air through your water before use. You can do this easily by shaking it vigorously.

The 3D shape should NOT sit in water. As long as moistness is high, you can spray with the 6.5 pH solution two times per day for the first two days, at that point once every day until it roots. Be that as it may, the moistness must be high; you should see condensation inside on the plate walls and perhaps the leaves. I also spray the walls of the plate to keep it damp. Spray just the leaves not the cubes.

Remember that the more you have damp conditions the almost certain it is to get shape or fungus; rooting rapidly is one approach to maintain a strategic distance from protracted moist conditions.

Water must be given by plant's leaves and the cut stem until roots can supply it. When watering your rooting medium make a point to keep the surface uniformly moist, taking special consideration not to over-water and suffocate your poor plant's recently forming root system. Water as expected to keep the develop medium uniformly moist and never let it get soggy.

WARNING: DO NOT over-water your precious clones! Keep the medium equally moist. You don't need it to get soggy or suffocate your roots.

Check for roots around the eighth day by opening a 3D shape down the middle cautiously. White roots should be exiting the hub.

How do I know if the rockwool cube requires watering?

To get watering of rockwool cubes absolutely right, use scales. Gauge a dry solid shape. At that point, saturate a shape and gauge it. Subtract the heaviness of the dry 3D shape from the wet one. You presently realize how much water is in the block when completely saturated(1g=1ml). Your 3D square needs water when weight drops to 20-40% of saturated weight. When you have done this a couple of times, you will have the option to estimate the weight and requirement for water by feel.

When using this methodology with clones, you'll need to guess the heaviness of the clone, perhaps 10-25g depending on the size of the cuts. When weighing a 3D square with a clone, subtract the estimated clone weight and dry solid shape weight based on what is measured to closely estimate water accessible in the block.

In most cases, especially when using a seedling warming mat, they will require water once at regular intervals. Cubes should never totally dry out.

Watering The Individual Cubes

Immerse the shape most of the way into a basin of pH adjusted (5.5-6.5) water for a couple of moments. Tenderly shake out (yet don't squeeze) excess water.

Rooted clones (roots are showing from the solid shape) should get completely soaked for around fifteen seconds, as they have the ability to take-up water quickly and will use that amount in twenty-four hours. Unrooted clones should just get a little plunge; three-five seconds all things considered. Key: Moist is superior to saturated for encouraging root development.

Try not to allow cubes to stand in water. In the event that excess water drains into the plate they sit in, void it out.

Start high nitrogen nutrients when roots have risen up out of the base of the shape – ¼ strength for first four to five days, ½ – ¾ the following four to five days, at that point maximum capacity from that point.

This strategy should give 85-100% success, with roots showing in five-seven days and profuse root advancement in ten days.

Stickiness

When cloning it is critical to keep natural factors at ideal levels to ensure as close to a 100% success rate as possible. One of the most influential components of clone success to control appropriately is the mugginess, also known as moisture level in the air. Clones will root the fastest when moistness levels are at 95-100%for the first two days, and gradually decreased to 80-85% during the following week. Air should be around 70°F (21.1°C).

On the off chance that you need a successful harvest, it is strongly advised by numerous veteran growers to put your clones under a moisture vault (this will keep mugginess in and help stimulate root development extraordinarily) to retain high stickiness. Make certain to mist them much of the time with a spray bottle loaded up with distilled water, and evacuate the arch several times every day to ensure that they get fresh air. The reason you mist them frequently (yes, the tops included) is because these clones have no beginning root structure to supply water to the plant. At the point when the plants are shrouded in moist water they won't dry out fast because of the dampness you are supplying them while they begin to establish their delicate little root structures.

Note: If you are strapped for cash you can easily make your own dampness tent using hard plastic, plastic bags, or glass. It is best to get one that appropriately seals and retains moisture however for most extreme results.

Transpiration is the process wherein water and nutrients travel up the stem from the roots to the leaves, where they are used in photosynthesis. Tiny hairs called stomata (tiny breathing pores situated on the underside of the leaf) sweat out the moisture to allow the stream of nutrients to continue flowing. Wind aids in transpiration by blowing the moisture off the stomata, which is the reason the dampness vault is so significant.

Another approach to ensure the stomata is to spray a light wax onto the cuttings. This slows transpiration to the point where you do not require a top, and the waxy coating serves as a security against pests. I suggest you just have a go at using a dampness arch at first, as this wax technique can be somewhat precarious and an undesirable alternative for natural intended growers.

Evacuate the cover once per day and fan the cuttings with it for a couple of moments. Some growers like to cut small holes into the corners of the cover so that there is a little ventilation. Putting holes into the corners of the plate to also benefits by allowing for drainage if the plants become over-watered. The roots need oxygen to flourish and survive!

Leave the solid shape in a mugginess vault at around 80-85°F (26.6-29.4°C), with around thirty-fourty W/sq of fluorescent lighting on for twenty-four hours every day.

Heating Clones

Clones root best when the develop medium is hotter than the encompassing air temperature of the room. At the point when the medium is a couple of degrees hotter it increases the concoction action and hastens root arrangement. Growing medium should be 75-80°F (23.8-26.6°C), as this is best. Anything above 85°F (29.4°C) can be dangerous and hurt the plants. Heating mats assist dry with outing and warm the cubes.

Oftentimes here a heating cushion, heating cables, or an incandescent light bulb put underneath the rooting cuttings is used. You will need to keep the air temperature 5 to 10°F (- 15 to - 12.2°C) cooler than the medium. A warm growing medium combined with a cooler air temperature will slow diseases and conserve moisture levels.

Diminish Cutting Stress

By controlling light levels, mugginess and temperature, your main responsibility is to keep the sensitive cutting in a total state of lethargy. Cuttings with out roots are sensitive to stress. Each exertion should be made to minimize dissipation from the cuttings and stay away from extraordinary light and temperature levels. Keep stickiness as close to 100% as possible and maintain water and substrate temperatures at between 70-84°F (21-29°C). Cooler water will slow root development; hotter water will energize disease. The lower the stickiness level, the more water the plant will transpire, causing the cutting to use up stored nourishment for things other than root generation. It is critical to hold the leaves as lethargic as possible and license the cutting to use a greater amount of it's vitality on root improvement.

Preserving Clones in the Fridge

You can keep clones stored for later use for two or three months in a cool fridge, just soak them in chilly water and afterward transfer to a zip lock sack. Open the sack each week or so to allow fresh air in. You can also put them inside a sodden paper towel or material. Keep the temperature in your cooler above 40°F (4.4°C). Temperatures beneath this level may cause the plant cells to harm.

This can be useful for various reasons. It is possible for very small cultivators to develop without the use of mother plants. It is also possible to hold the males in reserve without wasting space or having to stress over dropped dust. Holding clones in the ice chest offers numerous new possibilities for testing a wide range of males, holding strains while evaluating, changing the manner in which you time your mothers, and so forth.

Clones that are stored in the ice chest this way actually root faster than nonfridged clones once they are expelled, to a limited extent of two or three weeks, when they will take more time to root and you may lose a couple.

At the point when they are expelled from the refrigerator to be replanted, make certain to recut the stem with a sharp perfect sterilized razorblade, blade, or X-Acto blade.

Another technique for preserving your clones is by purchasing a commercially accessible gel that will empower you to store your cut clones until required.

Yellowing leaves on unrooted clones can be from an excessive amount of light, or the stem may not be solidly touching the rooting medium. Mood killer any CO_2 until they root. An excess of fertilizer can shrivel or wither clones, plain tap water is fine.

Having Trouble Cloning?

Some varieties are easier to clone than others. There are Sativas that will sprout roots so easy, you can (almost) stick them in the ground and disregard em. However, at that point there are some early Indicas that you can infant and they will just sit there and starve to death. Here are some things to focus on.

Issue Cloning

Help the roots develop: Figure out where the roots will develop on your cutting before you actually cut it. Keep this bit of the stem dull for up to fourteen days by wrapping some tape around it. This is called *etiolation* and will empower rooting. Make the cutting with a sharp blacksmith's iron pruner or sharp pair of scissors, and sterilize them after each cut. A dull pruner will crush the stem and it will be more enthusiastically for the roots to frame. An extremely sharp edge will make an even cleaner cut, which will also help rooting, yet be mindful so as not to cut yourself. Attempt to make the slice at an edge to increase the surface zone it has to absorb water.

Air Bubbles: The plant needs air to enable the roots to frame, yet don't give any a chance to get in the stem. This will remove the slim activity and make the poor cutting work ten times harder. Promptly submerse the cut end in water or rooting solution to keep this from happening. You could even take it over to the sink and make a second cut under running water in case you're really stressed over it. Leave the cutting in the rooting solution for a day or something like that. On the off chance that you just leave it in the water, you may luck out and sprout some roots, yet they really need some oxygen. You can effectively give O_2 by air circulation or passively circulate air through by using an airy medium.

Something else that makes the cutting work harder is breathing itself. Utilize your plastic vault or dampness tent to confine transpiration and shield the medium from drying out. Another approach to restrain transpiration is to cut about half off of every pamphlet. You will still have the same number of leaves on the stem, however the surface region has decreased. This also helps control fungus by preventing the leaves from contacting the vault or the medium.

Lighting: The best possible lighting is also significant. Direct sunlight will warm the air in the vault excessively, however they're not going to root in obscurity either. Fluorescents are perfect for this. A HID is ok if it's not very close, or you could even give them a touch of indirect sun from a window in the event that you can keep them warm.

You have watched out for the pH and the notes, and you see it's starting to develop again, so its safe to assume that it has roots and you can evacuate the mugginess vault. Occasionally a cutting may shrink a little at first, however give it a mist and it should liven up. In the event that none of these tips help, either consider tissue culture or finding an alternate mother.

Wilting Clones

In the event that your clones are wilting ensure they are immovably seated in the medium. On the off chance that they are *too immovably* seated, you may have bowed or broken the stem and stopped water take-up. Ensure that the lights aren't excessively splendid, fluoros are all that is required. Next time, a hostile to ranspiration spray will significantly lessen wilting, they structure a waxy boundary that keeps water inside the cutting.

The cuttings might be excessively huge with an excess of leaf mass. You can trim off the half of the fan leaves to decrease region or take smaller cuttings.

What's more, make sure to screen closely the encompassing air temperature as anything above 80°F (26.6°C) is starting to get excessively hot and this will serve to quicken both transpiration and the drying out of your medium.

PREPARING BONSAI MOTHERS

The most significant process when selecting clones is to appropriately choose a mother plant. A Bonsai Mother is a female strain kept in the vegetative state, never allowed to flower. Female plants will create 100% females, all precisely like their mother. A Bonsai mother can be kept for several years, however, it is suggested to begin once more every year by seed in request to proliferate another fresh sound mother. You take cuttings/clones from your Bonsai Mothers. Take clones from mother plants that are in any event two months old. Plants that clone before two months may most likely grow unevenly and have excruciatingly slow development.

Any female plant can be changed over into a bonsai mother. She can be developed from seed or be a clone of a clone. The moms should be solid, pest/disease free and completely into vegetative development. Clones can be taken off moms as long as two weeks into flower; notwithstanding, these flowered clones experience reveg shock and are regularly hard to root. It is wise to keep several bonsai mother plants in the vegetative development stage for a consistent source of cloning stock. On the off chance that you need to ensure most extreme quality bud generation, at that point start new mothers from seed each year.

A typical secret cloning propensity among professional weed growers is to foliar feed the mothers with a recipe containing Nitrozyme kelp separate containing development hormones three-four days before cloning. This will energize mind-blowing lush and sound shoot development.

BONSAI MOTHER GROWTH TIPS

Lighting: Under twenty-four hours of constant light the mother will have an exceptionally hard time flowering, the downside being that the mother may become faster than necessary. Under eighteen hours of light and six hours of darkness (generally alluded to as eighteen/six) that plant will have much slower development, the plant will get a decent rest period, and you get a lower electrical bill. The downside of eighteen/six is that sensitive strains may begin to flower or possibly produce pre-flowers, especially if the mothers are kept for significant stretches of time. Some strains are increasingly inclined to flower.

Generally unadulterated sativas require most extreme light in request to fool the plant into thinking it's summer, while stable indicas adapt better to eighteen/six. Going with a lower light system then eighteen/six should be considered test. 1200 lumens of blue spectrum rich light is bounty. You need to give mothers eighteen-twenty-four hours of light for each day to maintain fast and vigorous development.

Note: Always start with the best mothers you can find.

Nutrients: While the plant is dynamic in vegetative development stage, feed it with a decent quality, all-purpose or high Nitrogen fertilizer. Multi week before taking a cutting feed the Bonsai Mother plant with a low nitrogen, high Phosphorus flowering fertilizer. Lower nitrogen promotes rooting in clones, so around multi week before you take your cuttings lower it. Decrease the sum/proportion of Nitrogen in the mother's supplement solution three days before cloning (flush soil mothers with water). Nitrogen inhibits root development;

decreased N levels in the mother help the clones to root faster.

The flowering fertilizer will bring down the measure of stored nitrogen in the plant and increase the measure of stored carbohydrates necessary for the creation of roots. Spraying the foliage with water day by day will help quicken this process.

Taking Clones From A Flowering Plant

In the event that you take clones during flowering, the clones will take in any event two weeks to start vegging again. It may also take a couple of more weeks for the buds to be reabsorbed. During this time root development is frequently painfully slow. Since you've never harvested any buds from these clones future yield won't be compromised.

You should anyway not trust that clones taken from a flowering plant will survive, because clones taken from a flowering plant generally won't survive – in the event that you don't have the foggiest idea what you are doing and know your strain then you are gambling. It is prescribed to take clones just from plants in Vegetative Growth.

Since a cutting taken while the stock plant is flowering should be compelled to return to a vegetative state under a twenty-four hours light, this causes extra stress, slowing development and advancement. Rooting may occupy to three times longer when the cuttings are taken during the flowering cycle. The cutting might not have enough stored nutrients or carbohydrates to survive. In the event that you must do this, at that point take the cutting when the mother plant is just up to fourteen days into flowering.

Some growers don't care to top their moms, preferring to take clones from lower parallel branches to maintain vertical development and forestall bushy development. Topping will create two additional shoots at the same hub, and considerably more clones can be taken the following round.

What number of Clones Should I Cut?

There will always be regular differences between clones. Clones taken in huge numbers will compensate for poor performers and mortality. The fastest rooting clones have the most vigorous vegetative development and usually the best flowering potential. Taking roughly half more than you need is a decent starting point.

When Exactly to Take Cuttings?

Despite the fact that cuttings can be taken whenever in a plant's life cycle, the best time to take them is before the plant is flowering. This helps the cutting to root all the more easily. Numerous growers will develop out a plant until it has started to develop internodes, at that point they take their clones and discard the plant.

Unending Harvesting

Profitable growers have two develop rooms! One for vegetative development/cloning, and the other devoted for flowering. Business growers combine eight-week flowering/harvest cycles with continuous cloning to frame what is known as an *unending harvest*.

A model is to take two clones like clockwork, and harvest one ready female each other day. This way, every time a plant is harvested, a couple rooted clones are moved from the vegetative room into the flowering room. The above model will yield the producer thirty flowering clones that are on a ninty-day schedule. This means it will require some investment a clone is cut from the mother plant until the day it is harvested. On the off chance that this schedule was used, the cultivator would have thirty clones, ten vegetative plants and thirty flowering plants growing perpetually consistently.

The key of course is to have a separate veg and flowering chamber going at the same time. Each time a plant is harvested it gets supplanted with a clone from the veg room, so that the bud chamber's always completely filled.

Eventually, as you become familiar with the flowering times and cloning times of your strains, you can close in on the objective of 100% occupancy(with no additional clones laying around and no spot to put them). This does take a bit of calculating, yet once done you can jump on a fairly precise schedule to where you are picking your buds as expected. It's the perfect setup for growing various strains with various flowering times.

Hydroponic/soil systems: Since the plants will be of varying sizes, you will need a hydro or soil system that is helpful for moving them around under the lights, to keep them in that bowl development (or, in case you are vegging under fluorescents, in a staircase course of action with the lights hanging diagonally). You need it to be easy to position the plants any place you need in the chamber, plus be capable take them to the following chamber. Great systems include ebb/flo and drip, and furthermore soil/pots. Systems with fixed plant spacing (air and nft tubes) or potentially systems where the roots intertwine may demonstrate troublesome in a consistently changing ceaseless harvest setup.

An extraordinary plant can be restored and cloned considerably after it has flowered and been harvested.

On the off chance that a small measure of vegetative issue is left growing on the base of the plant and it is put under an eighteen hour light cycle then all the little nuggets will stretch into vegetative shoots, which may then be cloned and developed into a full mother plant, which can be cloned indefinitely. This will give you many uniform harvests of your preferred plant. This means you wont need to continually purchase seeds.

Cloning Technique

Cloning TechniqueThere are several methods of taking cuttings from your selected parent plant. The techniques with the most success rate and easiest to do will be outlined in this section.

Successful cloning requires cleanliness, warmth, sound stock, and a little care. Clones are sensitive to their condition. Harsh conditions (ie. unpleasant cold) will defer rooting and increase death rates.

Prior to Beginning

Before you begin cloning in request to ensure as close to a 100% success rate as possible please survey the following suggestions:

•	Select a strong solid female mother plant (*Bonsai Mother*).

•	Wash your hands completely in advance.

•	Keep your work territory, tools, and work surfaces spotless and sterile. (You can sterilize tools such as a razor, sharp scissors, x-acto blade and so on by dipping them in liquor or vinegar. Blanch that is weakened to a 5-10% solution also works wonders.)

• 	Have your pH adjusted develop medium prepared for prompt planting.

• 	Be sure to have all your cloning supplies in reach and promptly accessible before you start to take clones.

Taking Cuttings Using Rockwool

Rockwool is an astounding mechanism for cloning: sterile, modest, biodegradable, and convenient – rockwool can be transplanted into any system with minimum transplant shock.

Required Materials:

• 	Rooting gel/hormone.

• 	Fresh sterile razor blade(s)/quality trimming scissors.

• 	Cutting board.

• 	1″ rockwool cubes.

• 	Slotted plate/solid plate/High cap dampness domes.

• 	Flourescent lighting.

• 	Optional Materials:

• 	Heating mat.

• 	Isopropyl liquor.

• 	Tray inserts (to keep cubes upstanding, equitably spaced, and slightly raised off

• 	the slotted plate).

Note: always use *excellent water* when watering clones – distilled, reverseosmosis (RO) *or twenty-four hours* tap water left for twenty-four hours to dissipate chlorine. All water should be at room temperature.

Prepping The Rockwool

The first step is to treat the rockwool by soaking medium-term in a pH treated solution:

Step 1. Expel plastic wrapping from cubes (The plastic can incubate green growth)

Step 2. Set up some pH 5.5 – 6.5 water.

Step 3. Immerse cubes for twenty-four hours.

Here you can use plastic inserts to keep cubes upstanding, equally spaced, and slightly raised.

Many find the standard 1″ 3D square too huge; it remains soggy and cool (even on a heating mat). A superior thought is to cut the 1″ 3D square into two halves; the ½ sized block dries out faster, stays warm, air can arrive at all sides, roots exit faster, and you get twice as many. Cutting a 3D shape into four makes considerably more.

Note: Labeling your mother and the clones taken from a specific mother plant is a smart thought to backtrack on a *monster mother*.

Preceding cloning exposed clones will wither within a few moments, so it is best to have all materials prepared before you start to take cuttings:

- Dunk scissors and extremely sharp steel into liquor.
- Wipe cutting board with liquor.
- Drain cubes, place into plate.

- Jab a 1/8″ gap most of the way into the focal point of each 3D square.

Spread prepared cubes with vault until you are prepared to start(prewarming the rockwool by putting the filled plate on the heating mat for ½ hour before you start to take cuttings ensures a damn-close to 100% success rate).

CHOOSING CLONES

Effectively growing tops are liked, as they contain the most development hormones. Clones brought let down are regularly spindly and less created. The best is 3″ top clones with a 1/8″ stem, two-three fan leaves and a slightly firm (yet not yet woody) stem.

Short clones are best (close to two-three nodes), otherwise the recently forming roots must support a huge leaf and shoot. The clone should also be *develop*, with alternating leaves. Juvenile clones have leaves opposite one another and are usually pale and spindly.

Stay away from stem cuts (no hub) and fitting cuts, as they don't root so well (roots structure essentially at the nodes). Trim huge fan leaves into equal parts to minimize the leaf region the recently forming roots must support.

Selecting The Clone – Where do I cut?

Select a vigorous growing top on the mother, cut the main stem just over a fan leaf/assistant shoot hub around two nodes down. The cut should be possible with sterilized trimming scissors or an extremely sharp edge.

Leaving a shoot and fan leaf on the mother allows the remaining shoot to continue growing and another shoot to develop from that hub.

When taking a cutting you must slice it long enough to have at any rate one cut internode under the medium. Attempt to take a cutting that is at any rate three inches in length. When the cut has been made, trim off all leaves and branches with the exception of the best two fan leaves and the growing tip of the branch. This will leave a pleasant stem for planting. Ensure you use a sterile clean apparatus when making your cut.

An internode is the spot on the stem where the leaf (plus its stem) intersects the main stem. Cuttings taken from wood-like parts of the plants won't root as well as cuttings taken from the soft veggy part of the plant. Take them from the fresh soft parts to ensure most extreme rooting success.

The bigger branches of a cannabis plant will oftentimes have minimal white protrusions close to the base of the stem. These are known as *adventitious roots*. These most regularly will show up in a muggy situation and promptly develop into roots when set into a develop medium.

Cuttings taken from the lower branches are best as these regularly contain a higher measure of sugars and they root a lot faster than the slips from the highest point of the plant.

Note: Be fragile with your clones all through as long as they can remember cycle. Any kind of stress will significantly disrupt hormones and slow its development.

Pre-Trim The Raw Clone (Removing Lower Nodes)

When the growing top has been selected and cut from the mother, trim shoots and fan leaves from the lowest nodes. The lowest hub will be inserted into the rockwool.

Cut ¼" beneath the lowest hub with the extremely sharp edge at fourty-five degree point on the cutting board for a well put together.

Removing the huge fan leaves ensures that the delicate cutting's water and supplement take-up processes won't be overburdened.

The Trimmed Clone:

This *perfect* cut clone was taken from a vigorous top. A fan leaf and shoot were both expelled at the lowest hub. The clone will soon be inserted dunked into rooting gel/solution, at that point inserted into a rockwool 3D square.

Trim huge fan leaves down the middle. This will vastly influence improve your clone's initial advancement – (It reduces transpiration; so the recently forming roots don't need to initially support as a lot of leaf matter.)

Planting The Clone

Before placing your cutting in a medium if should be treated in a rooting solution such as fungicidal-b[1] blend, or the incredible Willow Water as described beneath. Rooting solutions advance solid root development which is an essential building hinder for growing damp, substantial sensational buds.

WARNING: An embolism may shape in your stem (an air bubble) in the event that you lay your cutting down on a counter before placing it in a develop medium. It is advised to take your cuttings just under tepid water. This will expel the possibility of an embolism forming. An air bubble inside your stem will stop liquid take-up and slaughter your clones. The best method to forestall this is directly subsequent to taking your cutting to promptly dunk them into your develop medium or water. This will keep air from getting caught in the empty stems.

Plunge the cut clone into the cloning gel/rooting solution, making sure the lowest hub is also thinly covered with gel. Expel any excess on the cut surface itself (so the cutting does not suffocate).

Tenderly push the stem into the rockwool. On the off chance that the gap is too huge, delicately squeeze the rockwool around the stem to seal it.

Vault and Lighting

Spray inside of moistness arch with No-Damp solution or similar, you can simply mist them. Try not to spray clones legitimately, as this can support fine buildup.

Pivot edge clones to keep their leaves inside of the plate. Spread the freshly cut clones with the vault.

Put the clone plate + arch under *warm white* fluorescent lights (sensitive unrooted clones require low light levels at first. Try not to blast them with direct HID lights or direct sun just yet!!).

The dampness arch should be left on for three days, lifted day by day for air trade. On the fourth day prop up the vault ¼" (slightly) on one side to adapt them (if wilting occurs, leave arch on for one more day and attempt again).

On the fifth day expel the arch. Roots should begin to leave the 3D square following ten days or somewhere in the vicinity.

On the off chance that the lower leaves start to turn yellow and kick the bucket, do not stress that is flawlessly ordinary. It is simply the plant feeding off to sustain life by moving significant supplement and water from the more seasoned development. Try not to expel any dead development until the plant is very much rooted. On the off chance that you evacuate the dying development the plant can starve and pass on totally. At the point when the clone has created roots, replant it where you need it.

Every day Maintenance

Air trade: Lift the arch in any event once every day (for first three-four days, at that point expel vault). Here is a little stunt; breathe out inside the arch to increase CO_2 levels. As the Native Americans say, when we breathe out, the plants inhale.

Watering: Water each second day when the clones are under the arch, at that point once/day from that point. When roots show, you may need to water two times per day to keep the roots moist.

The pH of the water inside of the rockwool will rise slowly; re-hydrating at 5.6-5.8 will restore legitimate pH levels inside the root zone. Allowing the cubes to dry slightly will compel roots to search for water and support vigorous rooting (yet dont allow the cubes to totally dry out!)

Blend 5.6-5.8 pH *twenty-four hours* water and fill solid plate most of the way with water.

Note: After the vault has been evacuated, include small amounts of nutrients.

Plunge clones + inserts + slotted plate into the ½ filled solid plate. Ensure all clones are getting water by *swirling* the edges of the plate.

Lift clone plate out and allow to drain. Shake plate to evacuate excess moisture. Spot clones back under fluorescent lights, and a delicate fan.

Root Check

Roots should begin to leave the shape in seven-ten days. A delicate upward pull on the clone will let you know whether it is rooted (just do this following ten days). Unrooted clones will haul out. Roots might be present, yet not yet exiting the block. If all else fails, cautiously open the solid shape to see if any roots are exiting.

Initially clones will draw their supplement needs from the fan leaves, and may turn slightly pale. This is a decent sign, as it is verification the clone is rooted, and is effectively growing. Regularly unrooted clones seem solid and green (and will stay that route for weeks).

To make things easier, you can sort out the clones (unrooted, hardly any roots, vigorous) into their own trays. Roots should be white and fluffy. On the off chance that a clone has not shown roots in two weeks, I'd consider removing it. Dark colored roots indicate decay, and nature is beginning to restore your plant over into the soil. (It's dead.) Occasionally, root tips will become air consumed: a sign to water all the more frequently!

Powerless nutrients (50-200ppm) should be started on the rooted clones, and watered all the more every now and again to abstain from drying the exposed root tips out. You could also attempt a powerless foliar feeding with any kelp separate. Gradually begin to increase Nitrogen levels.

Once Rooted

At the point when you first see the cutting is rooting through the solid shape base, you can stop spraying and start watering the 3D square, and let the solution drain from the 3D shape.

This is a crucial time:, when you see roots, water the solid shape and open the tent a little to allow moistness to escape and check at regular intervals for ANY sign of wilting. In the event that after the first hour with no wilting open the tent somewhat more, and check each hour. Following four to six hours with no wilting, you're prepared to shake n' roll.

In the event that any clones start to wither supplant the tent, spray leaves, and attempt again the following day. On the off chance that you have some rooted, some not, go for the moistness for a couple more days.

When the clones have completely established roots, they can be put under powerless HID light and a frail (250-500ppm) supplement system, or outplanted into soil, hydro or aeroponic systems. Clones are allowed eighteen-twenty-four hours of light so that they stay in the vegetative development stage. Clones generally will take ten-twenty days to grow a strong sound root system. When the root system is established, clones are transplanted into a bigger container or develop medium.

Presently they are prepared to develop for one-four weeks in the vegetative development stage before they are compelled to flower.

Tips

•   Do not put the clone plate legitimately onto a heating mat. The warmth will cook the roots, even on a clock. It is smarter to raise the plate off the tangle. A coroplast strip or two to sit the plate on works extraordinary raising the plate approx. ¼".

•   A low-level continuous warmth is liked, yet a clock might be required to lessen temperatures. Running your mats thirty minutes on, thirty minutes off, every minute of every day is immaculate. In any case, keep close watch, the warmth will dry out the clones, and incessant watering might be required.

•   Occasionally, fresh cloning gel will be thick. Add some water to container, shake. The gel should pour easier.

•   If you are using rooting powder, take care to expel excess powder from the stem cut as you plant the cutting, as this can inhibit the take-up of water.

•   Give your rooted clones a foliar feeding with any Kelp concentrate to give them a brisk development boost.

•   Cut numerous tops without a moment's delay to speed up the cloning process.

Check and date all trays, so you realize when to anticipate roots. Attempt to keep various strains composed in their very own trays, watered separately.

Use a fresh blend of nutrients, and keep the jug sealed. pH can shift radically, yet usually wont do as such for the first ten days if the container's kept sealed, out of light, and at room temperature.

Albeit most clones will be prepared to plant within ten-fourteen days, you can keep them for quite a long time if need be by utilizing certain preservation methods(discussed beneath).

What's more, remember HUMIDITY, HUMIDITY, HUMIDITY. Be that as it may, do not try too hard for a really long time or you risk form and damping off.

TIPS TO MAKE BUDS BIGGER DURING FLOWERING

The most foreseen stage of a cannabis plants life is when buds start to show up.

What's more, every cultivator wants the largest, juiciest buds.

SEVEN TIPS THAT WILL SHOW YOU HOW TO MAKE BUDS GREATER DURING FLOWERING.

How To Make Buds Bigger During Flowering

Buds are the piece of the cannabis plant that contain the highest levels of THC, the psychoactive intensify that gives you that exquisite 'high' feeling.

Buds also contain other significant cannabinoids used for medicinal purposes such as CBD, THCV and CBG. So we need them as large as possible.

Before we begin, it's significant that you understand the basics of growing weed.

Numerous things can affect your yield before the flowering stage. Nonetheless, picking a High yield strain, using a fair LED develop light together with the effectively sized develop tent will have the biggest positive impact on your yield.

In case you're certain you have the correct set up, here are 7 tips on the most proficient method to make buds greater during flowering...

1. Increase Your Light Intensity

Increase Your Light Intensity How To Make Buds Bigger During Flowering. I'm sure you're mindful that when all is said in done, all the more light generally means a bigger yield.

The most successful step you can take to increase the size of your yield is to push the farthest point of light intensity that your plants are receiving.

Cannabis is a strong plant, and can actually absorb a surprising measure of light without harm.

You should in this way be as aggressive as possible when choosing the distance between your shade and light. For LED develop lights, you should drape your light somewhere in the range of 12" and 18" over the covering when flowering.

The ideal distance will fluctuate from light to light, so It's significant you consult the manufacturers instructions and test the light at various heights.

Start at 12 inches, at that point watch out for your plants throughout the following twelve hours and search for signs of light consume, which is a sign that your lights are excessively close. On the off chance that they are, inch them back until the light consume stops.

For ideal yields, you have to drape your light at the distance just before light consume occurs.

2. Dull means dim!

Cannabis starts budding when plants get in any event twelve hours of interrupted darkness every night.

After plants start budding, they must continue to get long dull nights until harvest or they may return to their vegetative state.

When the plant is changed to the flowering lighting schedule (twelve hours on, twelve hours off) there is generally another six-ten weeks before the plants buds are prepared for harvest.

It is absolutely essential to ensure that plants are not exposed to any light during their dull period, as they may return to vegetative development, severely limiting the size of the buds.

3. Ensure Air Circulation/CO_2

Once your develop lights are upgraded for intensity, you have to ensure your plants can inhale appropriately. Your cannabis plants require CO_2 as a component of the photosynthesis process, when they convert usable light into vitality.

Without CO_2, your plants would shrivel up and bite the dust. Plants can absorb A LOT of light before they require CO_2 supplementation. Along these lines, for most growers, a simple rotating fan will be sufficient to flow the air and give plants enough CO_2 to process the light.

4. Pruning

Pruning is a strategy that most growers use to increase their yield. The small shoots between the main stem and the branches are expelled so that vitality is redirected to flower creation.

You should just do any pruning during the vegetation stage of development, as the plant will require sufficient time to recoup from the shock and resume development.

Ensure your plants are growing again and evaporating enough water.

Abstain from adding any extra fertilizer until they are showing signs of recuperation.

5. Dispose Of Any Male Plants

Cannabis plants have two pairs of sex chromosomes, one of which carries the genes that determine sex (male or female). On the off chance that you are growing non-feminized seeds, each sex has a half possibility of occurring.

On the off chance that your plants are not developed from clones, you must sex your plants. Sexing your plants and removing the males will ensure that cross pollination does not happen.

By getting free of the male plants from your nursery, this allows the female plants to develop enormous and seedless buds, alluded to as sensimilla.

A cannabis plant won't start to show its sexual orientation until it enters the pre-flower stage. This can happen as ahead of schedule as three to six weeks into the plants life cycle.

When your plants are roughly three to six weeks old they will start to display signs of pre-flowers, which will indicate the sex of the plant before it enters its flowering stage.

It is essential to evacuate male plants as soon as possible. Plants that don't uncover their sex at the pre-flowering stage will uncover their sexual orientation in the first one-three weeks after the lights have been switched to a twelve-twelve flowering cycle.

6. Adjust Your Fertilizer To Match Your Plants Requirements

By adjusting your supplement giving to your plants definite requirements, your plants will become the largest buds possible. It is significant not to overload them as an oversaturation of nutrients can hurt or even murder the plant.

During the vegetative stage of development, a multi-purpose fertilizer might be used. Cannabis plants respond well to a blend of fertilizer that is high in Nitrogen, Kalium (Potassium) and Phosphor.

Be that as it may, in the flowering stage, your plant needs fertilizer with a more significant level of Kalium (Potassium) and Phosphor, and low levels of Nitrogen. The reason is that Phosphor will stimulate your plant to sprout more buds while the Kalium (Potassium) increases density and weight. Ideally, you need to use a fertilizer that has been grown specifically for the flowering stage.

Check Your PH Level

On the off chance that you are fertilizing your plants, you must consistently screen the pH level of your growing medium. Without the right acridity level, nutrients won't dissolve appropriately and the cannabis plants root systems can't absorb them.

The ideal pH run for cannabis plants developed is soil is 6.0 – 7.0 and 5.5 – 6.5 for hydroponic setups and plants developed in coco peat.

7. Harvest At The Right Time

Picking the perfect time to harvest is imperative to the yield you will get. Leaving your buds to age completely could mean 25% more to your yield. By inspecting your plants trichomes closely, you will have the option to determine precisely when you're plants should be harvested for greatest yield and intensity.

Final Thoughts

During this book we have focused on the best way to expand bud size during the preflowering, or flowering stage of the pants life cycle. While the techniques listed above have been demonstrated to work, a definitive objective of any cannabis producer should be to become the healthiest plants possible and this covers everything from seed selection to address care during the significant vegetative development time frame.

By ensuring your plants are sound consistently, you are ensured an abundant harvest.

MOTIVATIONS TO GROW YOUR OWN WEED

Have you ever thought of developing your very own weed? Maybe you should. It holds numerous favorable circumstances over purchasing weed from the road, and making it a very satisfying encounter.

Choosing to dive in and develop your very own cannabis can be an extraordinary method to reduce expenses and increase a ton of power over what you smoke. Taking into account what number of individuals smoke weed over the world, just a couple of us attempt to really develop it. This implies except if you live in a more pot tolerant nation, for example, the Netherlands or Spain, you need to depend on underground market sellers to get a stockpile.

Developing your very own cannabis is a compensating experience, and not as a result of the item that outcomes from it. In case you're searching for some inspiration to begin your own marijuana garden,.

Here is our summary of the main ten motivations to become your own!

1. YOU WILL SAVE A LOT OF MONEY

Weed is costly when you get it, yet modest when you develop it. Contingent upon where you live, the expense per gram fluctuates a great deal, however, it positively isn't modest. Obviously there is nothing incorrectly supporting your neighborhood organizations, especially in the event that you have the benefit to live in a spot where it's legitimate is (or semi-lawful). Be that as it may, in the event that you might want to spare money, there's no chance to get around developing you possess.

What's more, don't feel that so as to develop weed you need a perplexing, costly, full-on develop room. Developing outdoors is the simplest: All you need is a seed, soil, water, and light - and nature gives a large portion of that to free.

2. YOU KNOW WHAT YOU GET

Probably the most serious issue with purchasing weed is that you never truly realize what is in it. Has it been showered with overwhelming pesticides? Is it sullied with bugs? Who knows? Your vendor is probably not going to let you know. By developing your very own you can sit back and relax realizing you have all out authority over what is utilized, and the general last nature of your bud.

It likewise offers you the chance to dry and fix your very own marijuana. Relieving cannabis is the way toward permitting the chlorophyll left in the bud to separate, and it drastically improves the nature of your weed - making for a much smoother smoke. The thing is, most normal weed you can get hasn't been appropriately relieved as it takes a long time. Be that as it may, when you had very much restored bud you will never come back, it is the thing that genuinely sets the imprint for some epicurean quality stuff.

3. YOU ARE SELF-SUFFICIENT

"Dope will get you through occasions of no cash superior to anything cash will get you through occasions of no blockhead." Unless you are fortunate to live in Amsterdam or Barcelona you in all likelihood won't have the option to pick bud from a menu, if there's any whatsoever, contingent upon your area. Almost certain, you rely upon what is on offer by companions and companions of companions. Also, you conceivably need to manage individuals you would preferably not.

At the point when you develop your own you can escape both trashy weed and times of no weed by any stretch of the imagination. Additionally, you don't need to make that suspicious telephone call.

4. YOU HAVE ROOM FOR EXPERIMENTATION

Developing your very own marijuana can yield a considerable amount of bud. Where you would regularly apportion the stuff you get off the road, you will probably wind up with all the more then you comprehend how to manage on the off chance that you develop it yourself. Indeed, even one plant can yield immense sums. This gives you more space for experimentation. You can deal with transforming those abundance yields into edibles (shouldn't something be said about Space Cake?), or a tincture for stealthy in a hurry dosing. Maybe you can begin fusing it into your cooking by imbue it is a few oils. The possibilities are boundless, and you will have the whole weed at needed to investigate everything.

5. YOU DEVELOP A RELATIONSHIP WITH THE PLANT

As a little something extra, there is fulfillment. To realize that you developed your very own bud from seed to complete with your very own hands and the exertion is gigantically fulfilling. It brings about you building up an a lot further association with your plants, enabling you to truly welcome the experience and final product significantly more.

Additionally, with each develop your expertise will improve. Developing cannabis is a consistent learning experience, and realizing your next bunch is probably going to be superior to anything the latter is an energizing prospect. You will in the end up as a specialist producer, ready to peruse your plants and increase a smart thought of their quality essentially by how they are developing. You will never purchase marijuana again.

6. MORE CANNABIS STRAINS TO CHOOSE FROM

On the off chance that you have a Cannabis Social Club or a dispensary close by, you are one of the fortunate ones that can browse a various menu of many energizing strains. On the off chance that you don't have that extravagance, you are subject to companions or much of the time the bootleg market, where you chiefly get one strain that is of modest quality. Once in a while, more than one strain is offered, however that is not the standard. Developing your very own gives you a lot of alternatives to look over. Most home cultivators develop more than one plant. Along these lines, you have the delight of smoking an assortment of cannabis strains with various impacts, fragrances and flavors. Since smoking a similar same again and again gets sort of exhausting after some time, isn't that right?

7. IT IS FUN TO GROW YOUR OWN MARIJUANA PLANTS

A frequently disregarded point is that developing your own reserve of weed is too fun. It is an incredibly energizing pastime and energy on the grounds that there is simply such a long way to go and attempt. Think about all the various strains, systems, developing techniques and styles, and hardware that you can explore different avenues regarding. It is truly remunerating to see the outcomes. Getting another developing technique right or developing another tasty assortment to its ideal will put a grin all over. It is fun, however you can be glad for yourself too.

8. DEVELOPING CANNABIS IS EASY

At the point when you read about developing cannabis, it now and then appears as though it's the most troublesome activity. In any case, have confidence, it is most certainly not! Particularly when you stick to simple to develop strains and apprentice arrangements that can be acquired as a total set. Obviously, there are many propelled methods and development styles yet you can get to those later. In any event, for a novice, extraordinary outcomes can be accomplished with next to no exertion. A few suggestions for simple to develop

184

strains to begin with would be Northern Lights, Easy Bud or Critical. These strains are known for being learner amicable, yielding a lot of fine buds to stir your excitement.

9. THE STIGMA AROUND CANNABIS IS FADING

Numerous individuals who need to develop their own bud waver in view of the wrongdoing of the plant in their nation. What's more, that is just right! We urge no one to violate the law, yet with changing enactment in numerous spots, the entryway is at last open to purchase a tent and a few seeds and begin. Sometime, legitimization, or if nothing else decriminalization, will go to your place, as well. Also, educating yourself and finding out about developing weed in advance to get an extraordinary beginning when it at long last is legitimate, there's nothing amiss with that, isn't that so?

10. YOU WILL HAVE A LOT OF LEFTOVER PLANT MATERIAL WITH ENDLESS POSSIBILITIES

As you may know, not just the blooms of cannabis can be used; the whole cannabis plant has something to offer for you. Be it leaves, trimmings, sugar leaves or even stems, they all contain cannabinoids (not as much as the blossoms, however) and can be utilized to extraordinary impact. Prominent utilizes are making edibles, tinctures, hash or in any event, rolling a leaf stogie.

The conceivable outcomes are practically huge, see? Thusly, you can up the advantages of developing your own cannabis considerably more and get an assortment of weed items. You will resemble your own dispensary!

GROWING TIPS AND TRICKS

A clone is a cutting off a plant that at last grows roots. When a root system is established, the clone would then be able to be planted to create another plant that is actually the same as the plant it was taken from. Knowing how to clone marijuana plants is just one more aspect of cannabis development. At the point when you realize how to clone weed, the entire growing match-up changes. Cloning gives you the chance to prop your preferred strain up for quite a long time and can significantly improve your chances of a successful harvest and overall yield.

For what reason do growers use clones?

Cannabis clones in a growClones are a path for growers to ensure that their plants develop at pretty much the same pace, going through each stage of their lifecycle at the same time. This is gigantically advantageous to growers and can significantly increase the success of one's harvest.

Knowing how to clone weed allows you to make indistinguishable replicas of your preferred plant on numerous occasions. Find a strain that you love? Cloning it lets you continue to appreciate it harvest after harvest. I've been talented a couple Bubblegum clones in the past that are reputed to have been circulating for a considerable length of time.

Learning how to clone your cannabis plants will take your development skills to another level completely. Peruse on to find out just how easy cloning weed can be.

When you have it down, cloning weed becomes like second nature. There are actually a couple of various methods of cloning. These include cloning in water, soil, and rockwool. Every technique is simple and what works best for you basically comes down to personal inclination.

CONCLUSION

Growing your own marijuana is actually easy. Sure, there are a ton of cutting edge techniques, and there is always something new to learn and master, however the basics are truly simple, and once you have them down, you can easily create your indefinite supply.

How your cannabis is developed is significant, and here at Grown Rogue, we pride ourselves on recognizing which strategy is fitting for specific strains. While growing methods are becoming even more a focus because of an increase in development operations, the driving power that determines what kind of cannabis an individual should search for at last depends on how individual strains, from which cultivators makes you feel. How can it smell? How can it taste? How can it make you feel? Be it indoor, outdoor, greenhouse, any of these methods may create your preferred marijuana.

Feminized medicinal cannabis seeds are specially developed for the medicinal cannabis user. Truth be told, all cannabis types are fitting for medicinal use. In any case, some types are progressively suitable because of the dynamic substances.

Cultivating cannabis from seed is a bet; not exclusively is the nature of the seed's genetics in question, yet how well it was preserved as well. On the off chance that you have been cultivating for some time now, ideally an extraordinary plant has risen. One from which the bud was so great, you could barely handle it.

You thought it was past your abilities to accomplish such a specimen, and you would prefer not to see it go. Imagine a scenario where you could get increasingly out of your proudest green accomplishment. There is, truth be told, an approach to keep those genetics around longer. Start our manual for maintaining your own *mother plant*.

Cannabis can be recreated asexually or sexually. Asexual proliferation is what is known as *taking cuttings or cloning*. Numerous growers exploit this awesome process known as cloning. Simply stated, the cloning process is when development shoots or branches are expelled from chosen contributor plants and induced to frame roots in a separate develop medium. By taking cuttings from a mother, each and every clone will be an ensured female plant. A nursery can be propagated indefinitely by taking cuttings before plants begin to flower.

To enable you to out, here are the cannabis seed banks that work in any nation.

Cloning offers growers numerous benefits. For one it allows them to have a constant supply of female plants — by using clones, a cultivator has a sound, steady supply of ensured female-just plants. A clone is a careful hereditary copy of its parent. So, you can use your most vigorous and strong plants to use as mothers, and each clone you take from it will be vigorous and intense as well! Clones will always keep the same sex and force of the mother plant. It is also possible to make a nursery of plants that will last for a considerable length of time through cloning from a single female *bonsai mother* plant.

Disclaimer

This book is not intended as a substitute for the medical advice of physicians. The reader should regularly consult a physician in matters relating to his/her health and particularly with respect to any symptoms that may require diagnosis or medical attention.

(health, Cannabis)

Do not go yet; One last thing to do

If you enjoyed this book or found it useful I'd be very grateful if you'd post a short review on it. Your support really does make a difference and I read all the reviews personally so I can get your feedback and make this book even better.

Thanks again for your support!